Bedside Guide for Neonatal Care

Learning Tools to Support Practice

Julia Petty

 macmillan education   palgrave

First published 2015 by
PALGRAVE

Palgrave in the UK is an imprint of Macmillan Publishers Limited, registered in England, company number 785998, of 4 Crinan Street, London, N1 9XW.

Palgrave Macmillan in the US is a division of St Martin's Press LLC, 175 Fifth Avenue, New York, NY 10010.

Palgrave is a global imprint of the above companies and is represented throughout the world.

Palgrave® and Macmillan® are registered trademarks in the United States, the United Kingdom, Europe and other countries.

ISBN 978-1-137-39846-8   ISBN 978-1-137-39847-5 (eBook)

DOI 10.1007/978-1-137-39847-5

This book is printed on paper suitable for recycling and made from fully managed and sustained forest sources. Logging, pulping and manufacturing processes are expected to conform to the environmental regulations of the country of origin.

A catalogue record for this book is available from the British Library.

A catalog record for this book is available from the Library of Congress.

Typeset by MPS Limited, Chennai, India.

Contents

LIST OF ILLUSTRATIONS

BOXES

TABLES

FIGURES

INTRODUCTION – THE A to Z OF NEONATAL BEDSIDE CARE

This guide has been devised as a quick reference bedside resource of useful learning tools relevant to the care of the neonate in the clinical setting. The purpose of this book is as a general guide for bedside care containing information to support practice for health professionals working with neonates in the hospital environment. It is not the intention of this book to give lengthy explanations or protocols, nor is it intended to replace approved polices or company equipment user guides. Rather, it is to offer a 'snap-shot' reference guide to support knowledge for bedside care with reference to relevant literature and national guidelines where applicable. In this way, the book aims to be universally applicable to anyone caring for neonates in the clinical setting.

It is acknowledged that local thinking and guidance will invariably affect certain practices, which may influence the applicability of certain parts of this guide at local unit level. Therefore, where necessary, reference should be made to any relevant local protocols or formal practice guidelines in one's own clinical area and workplace. Acknowledging the general guide offered by this book alongside one's own local variations hopes to make the book a contextual and relevant resource to support practice and learning.

However, while being mindful of one's own unit guidance, it should also be remembered that when local practice does differ from said book, this can actually provide an additional opportunity for learning and further discussion. Moreover, learning different practices can serve to move learning on from just knowing *local* practice and open up opportunities for readers to begin to question why these variations occur along with what effect they might be having on neonatal care and outcomes.

After all, health professionals should learn from each other across different disciplines or neonatal units. There is never usually only one way of performing practices and variations will always exist. The main message is that whatever specific guidelines are followed, we are all aiming for the same outcome; that of optimizing care and minimizing risk to our vulnerable neonates and their families.

Another point worth noting is the importance of recognizing the continually evolving nature of some aspects of neonatal care; for example, the debates around early or late cord clamping in the newborn, ventilation modes and feeding regimes. The reader will be alerted to such areas, where applicable, as well as to any other area of caution requiring specific attention.

The book is divided into two main sections. In Part 1, the book starts by introducing the concept and importance of bedside learning in neonatal care and places this in the context of the holistic care of the neonate and family.

A discussion on the application of bedside learning tools for neonatal practice then follows, addressing how learning tools can be applied to the clinical area within an evidence-based approach. Part 2 covers over 100 key bedside tools for neonatal care, which is divided into 24 chapters according to an A to Z approach. The focus is on information to support practice, rather than the relaying of information on the theory of neonatal conditions, although where applicable, suggestions for further reading are provided for those topics that have a body of underpinning theory. The specific detail and layout of each chapter will be explained in the next section, 'How to use this book'.

HOW TO USE THIS BOOK

The book is intended to support essential learning in neonatal nursing practice and it is therefore expected that the reader will take it to the bedside. The reader should familiarize themselves with the A to Z organization within Part 2; Key Bedside Tools for clinical neonatal care, in relation to the topics covered, as well as how the chapters are formatted in a consistent way.

Each chapter in Part 2 relates to a letter A through to X. Some of the chapters are further divided into sub-sections each with an introduction highlighting the importance and relevance of that topic to practice. The bedside tools then follow. To give consistency, the tools are in one of three formats, namely, summary tables, checklists and flow charts or diagrams that are labelled accordingly (see key overleaf). Where required, specific tools may have an introductory brief to guide the reader to their use in practice. In addition, for each one, a 'Stop and think' symbol and text box highlights important practice points of clinical significance or areas of caution. Cross-referencing between chapters, where applicable, is provided by frequent signposting, indicated by a 'signpost' symbol to direct the reader to related areas of practice. Each sub-section is supported with a brief topic-specific glossary of terms to explain any relevant neonatal condition and/or related pathophysiology in a concise way and, finally, a relevant evidence base. References support each unit and, for certain topics, a brief list of resources for further depth and reading into the underpinning theory is provided.

As stated above, in Part 2 the readers are reminded to refer to their own unit policies, a message that is threaded through the whole book. Although the information presented is designed to be as universally applicable as possible, it should be considered within the context of, and in conjunction with, specific local variations. Therefore, rather than trying to cater for all eventualities and variations which would be onerous and potentially confusing, a boxed space is provided at the end of each sub-section, where applicable, to remind the reader to check local variations and guidance with additional space to note their own personalized unit-specific details. Finally, another common alert for the reader that is relevant to all topics where clinical practices are performed is a reminder of standard precautions in line with prevention of cross-infection, again indicated by a symbol. The above-mentioned boxed spaces and alert symbols used in the book can be seen in the key overleaf.

KEY TO SYMBOLS USED IN PART 2

The figures used throughout the book are categorized into the following formats:

CHECKLIST

FLOW CHART OR DIAGRAM

SUMMARY TABLE

There is one box for each figure to highlight important points, cautions or areas of controversy.

Each sub-section ends with the following boxes and symbols:

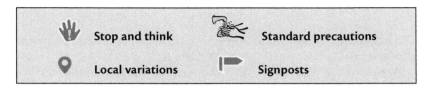

Stop and think	Standard precautions
Local variations	Signposts

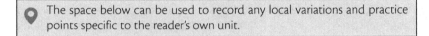

Where applicable, this symbol and box highlights important infection control reminders.

The space below can be used to record any local variations and practice points specific to the reader's own unit.

Links with related chapters and topic areas will be highlighted by this symbol throughout the book.

ACKNOWLEDGEMENTS

The author and publisher would like to thank the following publishers, organizations and individuals for permission to reproduce copyright material:

A. Mancini for Figure 2.31c 'Withdrawing or withholding treatment in the neonatal unit' from 'Practical guidance for the management of Palliative Care on neonatal units' (2014); Bart's Health Neonatal Unit, Royal London NHS Trust for Box 2.27a 'Calculating fluids and daily allowances', Box 2.32b 'Reducing TPN Formulas', Box 2.38a 'Double volume exchange transfusion (DVET): Nursing care guide', and Box 2.38b 'Understanding dilutional exchange transfusion'; BLISS for permission to reproduce material in Table 2.30 'Family-centred care principles' from THE BLISS Baby Charter and Care Standards; British Association of Perinatal Medicine (BAPM) for Table 2.26 'Levels of care (dependencies)' based on 'Categories of Care' (2010, 2011), Box 2.46 'Ethical-legal issues relating to parents in the neonatal unit', and Figure 2.31d 'End-of-life (palliative) care planning in the neonatal unit'; Elsevier for Table 2.1 'Guide for ETT sizing' from S. T. Kempley, J. W. Moreiras and F. L. Petrone 'Endotracheal tube length for neonatal intubation', *Resuscitation* 77 (3) (2008); Elsevier and Dr. J. Ballard for Table 2.5 'Assessment of gestational age' adapted from J. L. Ballard, J. C. Khoury, K. Wedig, L. Wang, B. L. Eilers-Walsman and R. Lipp 'New Ballard Score, expanded to include extremely premature infants', *Journal of Pediatrics* 119 (3) (1991); Emap Ltd for permission to reproduce Table 2.19 'Visual infusion phlebitis scale (VIPS)' from R. Higginson and A. Parry, 'Phlebitis: treatment, care and prevention' in *Nursing Times* (2011), originally from A. Jackson 'Infection control: a battle in vein infusion phlebitis', *Nursing Times* (1998); European Pressure Ulcer Advisory Panel (EPUAP) and National Pressure Ulcer Advisory Panel (NPUAP) (2009) for Table 2.34c from http://www.npuap.org/wp-content/uploads/2012/02/Final_Quick_Prevention_for_web_2010.pdf; *Infant Journal* and Louise Briggs for Table 2.34a 'Assessing tissue viability risk 1' adapted from C. Ashworth and L. Briggs., Design and implementation of a neonatal Tissue Viability Assessment Tool on the newborn intensive care unit 7 (6) (2011); *Infant Journal* and S. Lamburne for Box 2.9 'Nursing Care of the neonate on CPAP: specific practice points' from S. Lamburne, 'An assessment tool for infants requiring nasal continuous positive airway pressure', *Infant journal* 10 (4) (2014); Macmillan Publishers Ltd for Table 2.21 'Necrotising Enterocolitis and Bells (modified) staging criteria' from V. Lima-Rogel, D. A. Calhoun, A. Maheshwari, A. Torres-Montes, R. Roque-Sanchez, M.G. Garcia and R.D. Christensen, 'Tolerance of a sterile isotonic electrolyte solution containing select recombinant growth factors in neonates recovering from necrotizing enterocolitis', *Journal of Perinatology* 23 (3) (2003); MA Healthcare Ltd and Jane Willcock for permission to reproduce Table 2.34a (ii) adapted from J. Willock, M. M. Baharestani and D. Anthony, 'The development of the

Glamorgan paediatric pressure ulcer risk assessment scale', *Journal of Children and Young People's Nursing 1* (2007): 211–218; National Perinatal and Epidemiology Unit (NPEU) for Box 2.42a 'Therapeutic cooling criteria' and Box 2.42b 'Therapeutic cooling: nursing overview'; NHS Institute and Improvement and Dr Leonard colleagues for Figure 2.14 'SBAR(D) tool for communication and handover'; *Nursing Children and Young People* Journal for Figure 2.22a 'The metabolic triangle: the well neonate at birth' and 2.22b 'The relationship between the three Hs: compromise at birth' from M. Aylott 'The neonatal energy triangle part 1: metabolic adaptation', *Paediatric Nursing* (now *Nursing Children and Young People* Journal) *18* (6) (2006); Nutrition Care Pathway, East of England Perinatal Network (EEPN, 2012) for the risk categories and action in Box 2.33a 'Advancing enteral feeds in the at-risk neonate'; Springer Publishing Company for permission to reproduce Table 2.10 'A guide to ventilator modes', Table 2.11 'Ventilation parameters, useful formulas and definitions', Table 2.12 'Changing ventilation: a guide', Table 2.16 'Blood gas values', Box 2.10 'Setting a rate using inspiratory and expiratory times', Box 2.11 'A guide to weaning ventilation', and Box 2.13 'Interpretation of blood gases in the neonatal unit' from J. Petty, 'Understanding neonatal ventilation: strategies for decision making in the NICU', *Neonatal Network (4)* (2013); The Resuscitation Council UK for Figure 2.2 'The neutral position', and Figure 2.41 'Preterm baby in bag'; University of Wisconsin Hospital and Clinics for Table 2.31a 'Neonatal pain assessment tool 1: the Wisconsin scale for proverbal/nonverbal children' (adapted version) from http://prc.coh.org/pdf/Assess%20Cog%209-09.pdf; Wolters Kluwer Health, Inc. for Table 2.31b 'Neonatal pain assessment tool 2: COMFORT scale' from M. van Dijk, J. W. Peters, P. van Deventer and D. Tibboel, 'COMFORT Behaviour Scale: a tool for assessing pain and sedation in infants', *Am J Nurs 105* (1) (2005) and Oxford University Press as the original publishers for Table 2.31b 'Neonatal pain assessment tool 2: COMFORT scale' from K. Ambuel, K. W Hamlett, C. M Marx and J. L Blumer, 'Assessing distress in pediatric intensive care environments: the COMFORT Scale', *Journal of Pediatric Psychology 17* (1) (1992); Wolters Kluwer Health, Inc. for Table 2.31c 'Neonatal pain assessment tool 3: Preterm infant pain profile (PIPP)' from B. Stevens, C. Johnston, P. Petryshen, and A. Taddio 'Premature infant pain profile: development and initial validation', *The Clinical Journal of Pain 12* (1) (1996); UK National Screening Committee NHS Screening Programme for Figure 2.13 Heel prick correct position.

PART ONE – THE APPLICATION OF LEARNING TOOLS FOR NEONATAL PRACTICE

Neonatal care in context

Within the field of neonatology, nurses are a vital part of the multidisciplinary team (MDT) that provides care for sick neonates. The nursing care required by these neonates and their families in the hospital setting can be complex, meaning that there is much to learn for those working in this field. The past few decades have seen significant changes in the role of the neonatal nurse, along with considerable technological developments in neonatal units, changes in the education of neonatal nurses and ongoing clinical research activity within the speciality (Healy and Fallon, 2014). Not only have these advances in neonatal care made a meaningful contribution to the improvements seen in neonatal outcomes, but also the learning needs of nurses have become more diverse and varied (Petty, 2013, 2014).

The focus of this book lies in providing a guide for the clinical care of the neonate; i.e. that within the *hospital* setting. However, when caring for neonates in the clinical environment, fundamental care principles must not be forgotten in relation to treating them as individuals within a family care context. The following principles should be emphasized as being at the heart of caring for neonates and their families.

Fundamental principles of neonatal care

Firstly, neonatal practice is a *speciality*; that is, the specifics of the patient group and what is required for their care differs from that required for other patient groups. The unique anatomical and physiological features of the neonate, along with the smaller size and weight of the patient group, influences particular care practices. This can be illustrated with examples such as the interpretation of neonatal-specific blood value and vital sign ranges, the use of equipment designed around physiological norms and by the dosing, administration and metabolism of drugs. It is vital that anyone learning within this field captures the specific elements of the speciality.

Working within current neonatal care requires health professionals to acquire a sound repertoire of knowledge to support best practice for neonate and family. Learning resources, therefore, must be designed to meet the needs of the speciality and the related needs of the learner. Literature within healthcare on how best to support bedside learning suggests that health professionals require *discipline-specific* resources that are well designed and tailored to their learning needs (Sredl, 2006; Hyrkas and Rhudy, 2013; Petty, 2013). This book aims to provide such a resource in this speciality.

Secondly, one must remember that the *fundamentals* of care must never be forgotten regardless of how small and sick neonates are. Any neonate needs 'simple things done well' (Resuscitation Council, 2010) from the point of delivery into the world and for their ongoing care thereafter. These needs include providing adequate hygiene, nappy and/or mouth care, ensuring they are comfortable and pain-free at all times and remembering a humanistic, holistic approach to care. Although the book focuses on hospital-based or clinical tools in the main, the aim of neonatal care is to ultimately 'normalize' their care as soon as is appropriate and to get the family home.

The neonate as an individual

The neonate, like any service user of the healthcare system, should be respected as an individual, which includes their physical, psychological, emotional, social, spiritual and cultural needs. Care must be *culturally sensitive* (Flacking et al., 2012), recognizing diversity of ethnic background and religious observances of the whole family. In addition, neonatal care comprises that delivered to a range of different conditions and gestations; this book does not cover these individual conditions as it is intended as a general bedside guide that is universally applicable to any neonate. However, the delivery of interventions must consider the neonate's individual gestation, age, underlying condition and family context to tailor care most appropriately.

The neonate within the family-centred care context

It should be emphasized that any individual, specific care practice must be delivered within a holistic mindset, considering the needs of the neonate and the family as a whole. Family-centred care should always be at the forefront of neonatal practice. According to the Nursing and Midwifery Council (2010), family-centred care recognizes that, in most cases, children of any age, including neonates, are best cared for by their parents or certainly in a partnership approach between healthcare professionals and parents/carers. This partnership approach should include planning of care, negotiation of who will give that care and how primary carers for that neonate can participate as much as possible. The topic of family-centred care in practice will be covered later within this book in Part 2 (Key Bedside Tools for Clinical Neonatal Care). With the above concepts in mind, we must still remember that learners caring for neonates and their families must be equipped with the essential tools and vital information to do their job properly and safely, in order to ultimately deliver best practice to family units. This book aims to impart that information within this overarching context.

Bedside learning tools in context

The application of learning tools to neonatal clinical practice

A learning tool can be defined as something that a learner uses to work through concepts or processes while demonstrating his or her thinking, planning and/or decision making on the way to understanding and consolidating knowledge, in this case for nursing practice. Different formats for learning tools exist. However, the following features can be inherent in *any* learning tool, with examples from the author's experience, recognizing that not all tools will satisfy all definitions.

- Include customized steps to help learners perform a task or care practice; for example, a resuscitation *algorithm* or a *care pathway* for feeding. Similarly, *flow charts/diagrams* can provide building blocks that enable learners to step through difficult concepts or processes to reach predetermined learning goals; for example, a ventilation weaning flow chart or blood gas analysis. *Formulas* such as that used for drug and infusion calculations can also be classed under this category.
- Create and present observable points of knowledge or practice points; for example, an admission checklist or a pain assessment tool.
- Clarify what learners know and do not know; for example, a summary table that highlights the main points of a complex care practice such as ventilation practice or feeding. This can help learners grasp knowledge in a new area.
- Focus learning and help support learners as they work towards learning about a specific model of care; for example, a summary or checklist to provide an overview of the principles of developmental care or a charter for family-centred care bringing together the key components.
- Add to the meaning, linking the learning from the classroom to the clinical practice area; for example, applying the neutral thermal environment chart to set an incubator temperature ready for a neonatal admission.

With all this in mind, this book uses three overarching formats: Flow Charts/Diagrams (labelled Figures), Checklists (labelled Boxes) and Summary Tables, which fit in with the above-mentioned learning features. The three formats can be defined as follows:

- A *flow chart* is a sequence of steps, which represent actions in a particular process or activity. They are a type of *algorithm*, which can include a process for decision-making options or an ordered sequence of steps for a given practice. *Diagrams* are variations of flow charts and can appear in many different designs or formats, as applicable to the topic in hand.

- A *checklist* is a list of items, facts or names to be checked or referred to for comparison, identification or verification. This can include assessment tools.
- A *summary* (in the form of a look-up table) gives a brief account of the main points of a topic in a consolidated format.

Whatever format of learning tool is used at the bedside, the aim is that they are easy to use, accessible and concise, particularly for health professionals in a learning capacity, to aid and support optimum understanding.

The use of learning tools to support clinical decision making

Nurses and other health professionals perform a range of essential tasks and engage in key decision making in the bedside care of the neonate. To reiterate the point made earlier, neonatal care is a speciality that often requires health professionals new to the field to acquire a different and discipline-specific set of skills and knowledge to support their practice. Student nurses may attend the neonatal unit as a practice placement during their training programme, for example. Newly qualified nurses may then gain employment on a neonatal unit following registration, having gained varying amounts of neonatal experience during their training. Similarly, nurses from other fields may choose to work in neonatal care following a change in career path. Therefore, it follows that these individuals will require support with learning for effective decision making using appropriate tools. Whatever the reason for working in neonatal care, these nurses are faced with acquiring new knowledge within the remit of a beginner with limited experience in the field who uses taught general rules to help perform tasks. This 'novice nurse' learns differently and engages in less complex decision making than those who are more experienced and move from advanced beginner through proficient to expert level (Benner, 1984).

In practice, expert nurses collect a broader range of cues in the assessment of patient status than novice nurses (Hoffman et al., 2009). It is also well documented in the nursing literature that decision making among novice nurses tends to be linear, based on limited knowledge and experience in the profession and focused on single tasks or problems (Benner, 1984). As they make decisions, novice nurses are more likely to respond by using theoretical knowledge and psychomotor skills, rather than by engaging in more complex decision making (Gillespie and Paterson, 2009).

Furthermore, when novices lack experience in the clinical setting, they may rely on more experienced nurses until such a time as they become more competent and have sufficient experience to move to a more proficient and eventually expert level. This learning journey can take significant time and often, in today's healthcare climate, can occur with minimal support from experienced trained nurses who can be faced with a busy workload and limited time to teach. Therefore, it follows that novice nurses or other professionals in a learning capacity require access to learning resources to ensure their practice is safe and accurate, supported by clear information in an accessible format.

In clinical practice, nurses make numerous decisions throughout the course of a shift. Sub-optimal decision-making strategies may adversely affect the quality of nursing care provided (Twycross and Powls, 2006). It is imperative that nurses, whether they be novice or experienced are provided with the necessary tools to impart knowledge for safe practice.

It has been concluded that the nurse's awareness of the patient's situation, together with a well-founded basis for decisions provided by accessible and tailored information, can have positive effects on the nursing care provided (Hedberg and Satterlund Larsson, 2003).

Educators need to recognize that novices learn in a dependent fashion and that this type of learning is a natural process linked directly to their stage of role development. Educators can support novice learning by providing information, helping the novice set learning priorities and supporting them during the period in which they need to learn new and complex tasks.

Incorporating evidence into learning tools to support neonatal practice

The application of recent and valid evidence in the neonatal field is an essential part of delivering best practice to the neonate and the family. It is also integral to effective learning that knowledge is delivered and assimilated by the learner within the context of what the evidence has shown. The care provided by neonatal nursing is based upon scientific research and great strides have been made in translating research into practice in this speciality. Examples include the introduction of new ventilation techniques including non-invasive modes, the advent of surfactant and antenatal steroids in the light of evidence linking these to improved outcomes and the implementation of both developmental care and family-centred care principles into neonatal care delivery.

Learning tools therefore, should also have a grounding within this evidence-based perspective. Research has highlighted the benefits of, for example, learning tools that have incorporated recent evidence to guide specific care practices, such as, an algorithmic approach that can provide a step-by-step method for emergency care based upon evidence-based guidelines (Acquaviva et al., 2012). Evidence-based clinical practice guidelines include clinical protocols, care pathways and algorithms. Within these guidelines, researched statements supported by scientific literature should be subjected to regular multidisciplinary review reflecting current knowledge. Similarly, clinical or critical pathways provide a management tool which can help deliver standardized care. Clinical algorithms provide a flow chart of the process and those developed from an evidence-based perspective can facilitate the application of research to practice.

Interprofessional learning in neonatal care

Finally, it is important to remember that neonatal *care* is not delivered by nurses alone. Nurses caring for the neonate and family do so within a MDT perspective. Learning tools can be utilized by the MDT in relation to an interprofessional (IP) approach to learning in this field. This is congruent with the core essence of IP learning, which is seen as an essential component of current healthcare training and is relevant to a wide range of professions. The Centre for the Advancement of Interprofessional Education (CAIPE) states that, 'IP education occurs when two or more professions learn with, from and about each other to improve collaboration and the quality of care ... and includes all such learning in academic and work-based settings' (Barwell et al., 2013). Following on from this, learning tools that may benefit nurses may also be of use to the other members of the MDT. The neonatal MDT and the roles within this are covered later in Part 2 (Key Bedside Tools for Clinical Neonatal Care).

References

Acquaviva, K. D., Posey, L., Dawson, E. M., and Johnson, J. E. (2012). Using algorithmic practice maps to teach emergency preparedness skills to nurses. *Journal of Continuing Education in Nursing.* 43 (1): 19–26.

Barwell, J., Arnold, F., and Berry, H. (2013). How interprofessional learning improves care. *Nursing Times.* 109 (21): 14–16.

Benner, P. (1984). *From novice to expert: excellence and power in clinical nursing practice.* Menlo Park, CA: Addison-Wesley.

Flacking, R., Lehtonen, L., Thomson, G., Axelin, A., Ahlqvist, S., Moran, V. H., and Dykes, F. (2012). Closeness and separation in neonatal intensive care. *Acta Paediatrica.* 101 (10): 1032–1037.

Gillespie, M. and Paterson, B. L. (2009). Helping novice nurses make effective clinical decisions: the situated clinical decision-making framework. *Nursing Education Perspectives.* 30(3): 164–170.

Healy, P. and Fallon, A. (2014). Developments in neonatal care and nursing responses. *British Journal of Nursing.* 23 (1): 21–24.

Hedberg, B. and Satterlund Larsson, U. (2003). Observations, confirmations and strategies – useful tools in decision-making process for nurses in practice? *Journal of Clinical Nursing.* 12 (2): 215–222.

Hoffman, A., Aitken, L. M., and Duffield, C. (2009). A comparison of novice and expert nurses' cue collection during clinical decision-making: verbal protocol analysis. *International Journal of Nursing Studies.* 46 (10): 1335–1344.

Hyrkas, K. and Rhudy, J. P. (2013). Promoting excellence – evidence-based practice at the bedside and beyond. *Journal of Nursing Management.* 21: 1–4.

Nursing and Midwifery Council (2010). *Children's Nurses.* http://www.nmc-uk.org/Get-involved/Consultations/Past-consultations/By-year/Pre-registration-nursing-education-Phase-2/What-do-nurses-do/Childrens-nurses/.

Petty, J. (2013). Addressing learning needs in neonatal care: an overview of resources for self-directed learning. *Infant.* 9 (3): 102–107.

Petty, J. (2014). Exploring the effectiveness of an interactive, technology enabled learning tool to enhance student knowledge in neonatal biology. *Journal of Paediatric, Neonatal and Child Health.* 17 (1): 2–10.

Resuscitation Council (2010). *Newborn Life Support.* https://www.resus.org.uk/pages/nlsalgo.pdf.

Sredl, D. (2006). The triangle technique: a new evidence-based educational tool for pediatric medication calculations. *Nursing Education Perspectives:* 27 (2): 84–88.

Twycross, A. and Powls, L. (2006). How do children's nurses make clinical decisions? Two preliminary studies. *Journal of Clinical Nursing.* 15: 1324–1335.

PART TWO – KEY BEDSIDE TOOLS FOR CLINICAL NEONATAL CARE

DETAILED CONTENTS for A to Z (in order of appearance)

A   AIRWAY AND ASSESSMENT

Page no.

Airway management

Assessment

B   BREATHING AND BLOOD/BLOOD TAKING

Breathing and ventilation

Blood and blood taking

C   CARDIOVASCULAR CARE AND COMMUNICATION

Cardiovascular system (CVS) care

Communication

D   DRUGS AND DEVELOPMENTAL CARE

Drug administration

Developmental care

E   ENVIRONMENTAL CARE

F   FLUID BALANCE AND ELECTROLYTES

G   GASTROINTESTINAL CARE AND FEEDING

H   THE 3 H'S (METABOLIC TRIANGLE) AND HYGIENE NEEDS

The 3 Hs (the 'metabolic triangle')

Hygiene needs and care

I INFECTION AND IMMUNIZATIONS

J JAUNDICE

K KANGAROO CARE (SKIN-TO-SKIN)

L LEVELS OF DEPENDENCY

M MULTI-DISCIPLINARY TEAM (MDT)

N NEUROLOGICAL CARE AND NEONATAL ABSTINENCE SYNDROME

Neurological care

O   OXYGEN THERAPY

P   PSYCHOSOCIAL CARE OF THE FAMILY AND PAIN MANAGEMENT

Parents and family centred care principles

Pain management in the neonate

Q   QUALITY, RISK AND SAFEGUARDING

R   RENAL CARE AND RESPIRATORY DISTRESS

Renal assessment

Respiratory distress

S   SKIN CARE AND SURGICAL NURSING PRACTICE

Skin care and tissue viability

Surgical nursing practice

T   THERMAL CARE AND TRANSPORTATION OF THE NEONATE

The thermal environment

Transportation of the neonate

U   UMBILICAL CARE AND CATHETERS

V   VOMITING AND REFLUX

W   WEIGHT

X   X-RAYS AND IMAGING

Airway and assessment

This chapter covers two important topics in the immediate and ongoing care of the neonate: airway management and assessment.

Airway management

Ensuring a safe airway is an essential priority in any area of healthcare. This section focuses on useful tools in relation to managing the airway in the event of the neonate being unable to do so themselves. The majority of newborn babies breathe spontaneously within the first few minutes of life and open their airway adequately to ventilate and oxygenate themselves to sustain life after delivery. However, there are times in neonatal care when airway management is required for various reasons relating to the neonate's condition at birth or thereafter. This section starts therefore with a look at the principles of newborn and neonatal resuscitation, where maintaining a safe airway is absolutely essential to ensure safe outcomes.

> Related chapters: See *Assessment* which is a vital part of airway management along with *Breathing* and *Oxygen therapy* to view a range of tools to support care of the neonate requiring ventilation and oxygen respectively.

Preparing for resuscitation in neonatal care

Anyone who could potentially need to care for a neonate requiring resuscitation should be familiar with their own emergency trolley or Resuscitaire® along with the local procedure for checking equipment. Box 2.1 presents a checklist for what should be available on a Resuscitaire® and/or emergency trolley.

Box 2.1   Resuscitation equipment – CHECKLIST

- Attached to air/oxygen blender and gas source*
- Power source on* Overhead heater* Stop clock*
- T-piece connector and tubing connected to pressurized gas source, preferably with valve to give positive end expiratory pressure ('PEEP' valve)*
- Bag-valve mask (BVM) (for manual ventilation)

(continued)

- Two towels
- Stethoscope
- Face masks
- Suction catheters (wide bore: minimum size 10 fr)
- Laryngoscope with infant straight blade
- Oropharyngeal (Guedel) airways – 00 and 000 size
- Sterile endotracheal tubes (ETT) (of each size 2.5, 3.0, 3.5, 4.0)
- Sterile cord scissors and umbilical cord clamp
- Magills forceps introducer(s)
- ETT fixators
- Scissors
- Hats of varying sizes
- Plastic bags or plastic sheets (for preterm neonate)
- Umbilical venous catheters (UVC) and umbilical catheterization pack
- Sutures
- Emergency drugs: Adrenaline 1:10,000, Sodium Bicarbonate 4.2%, Dextrose 10%
- 0.9% saline for flushing drugs
- Syringes and needles
- Cannulas
- Nasogastric tubes
- Basic chest drainage equipment
- Non-sterile gloves
  Note: Items marked * are relevant to the Resuscitaire® only (see Figure 2.1)

📍 Check local guidance for any additional items that may be added

---

✋ **Preparation and equipment checking is essential at least on a daily basis to ensure readiness for emergency and unexpected events.**

Performing resuscitation at birth

A standardized approach is necessary for any resuscitation using a structured method to guide practice (Atkinson et al., 2010). The *order* of resuscitation is very important and reassessment for a response (increase in heart rate and visible chest movement) after *each stage* or intervention is essential in order to move on through the whole process. Box 2.2a–e depicts the Newborn Life Support (NLS) algorithm.

Figure 2.1   A Resuscitaire®

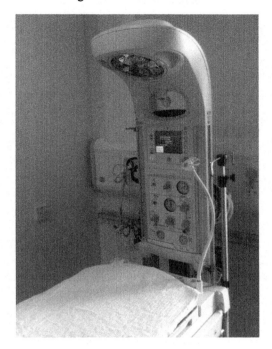

Figure 2.2   The neutral position

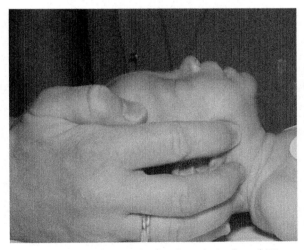

Source: Printed with permission from Resuscitation Council, UK

Box 2.2a   Newborn Life Support (NLS) – FLOW CHART

(Resuscitation Council, 2013)

Newborn baby at delivery
Dry the baby
(*exceptions apply (See Box 2.2b); for example, the preterm baby)

Remove wet towel and cover/keep warm
Start clock/note time/CALL FOR HELP
▽

Assess colour, tone, breathing and heart rate
▽

If not breathing
A Open the airway (neutral position – see Figure 2.2)
▽
If still not breathing

B Give 5 inflation breaths using air initially
(Add oxygen only according to pulse oximetry readings – see Box 2.2c)
(2–3 seconds each at pressure 30 cm/H_2O for term OR
* max. 25 cm/H_2O for preterm)

Look for a response (ask: has the heart rate increased? Is the chest moving?**)**

If no increase in heart rate, look for chest movement/CALL FOR HELP
▽
If no response

Recheck head position. Apply jaw thrust
Repeat inflation breaths. Look for a response
If no increase in heart rate, look for chest movement
▽
If still no response

Try alternative airway opening manoeuvres (see Box 2.2d)**/CALL FOR**
HELP

Repeat inflation breaths. Look for a response

If no increase in heart rate, look for chest movement
▽
Continue repeating inflation breaths UNTIL THERE IS A RESPONSE
▽
When the chest is moving

(continued)

Give ventilation breaths at 30/minute and check the heart rate
▽
If the heart rate is slow (<60/min) and not increasing

CALL FOR HELP
C Start good quality chest compressions immediately at ratio 3:1
(3 compressions to 1 breath) Place either both thumbs or two fingers just
under the nipple line. Press one third of the chest depth.

Reassess every 30 seconds looking for an increase in heart rate
D Consider venous access and drugs if no increase in heart rate
(see Box 2.2e)
▽
**If heart rate increases, stop compressions and continue ventilation
breaths at 30/minute until condition improves**

Box 2.2b   Exceptions to the standard NLS algorithm – SUMMARY TABLE

- Preterm neonates less than 28 weeks – place in plastic bag at delivery and
  dry head only, use less maximum peak pressure on inflation. In addition,
  preterm neonates are more likely to require oxygen.
- Presence of thick meconium in a neonate who is not breathing and unresponsive
  at delivery – suctioning under direct vision may be necessary *earlier than
  expected according to the above algorithm*; that is, as part of A, prior to B and C.

Box 2.2c   Normal oxygen saturation readings via pulse oximetry at birth

- Evidence recommends that resuscitation should be commenced using air in
  term newborns (Ramji et al, 2003; Tan et al, 2005). Oxygen is added *if required*
  as determined by pulse oximetry readings. **Acceptable pre-ductal oxygen
  saturations (SpO2) (via right hand) are;** 2 min 60%, 3 min 70%, 4 min 80%,
  5 min 85% and 10 min 90% (Resuscitation Council, 2013)

Box 2.2d   Alternative airway opening manoeuvres – SUMMARY TABLE

- 2 person jaw thrust, one to apply jaw thrust and the other to give manual breaths.
- Inspection of the oropharynx under *direct vision* and *suction only if necessary*.
- Insertion of an oropharyngeal (Guedel) airway under *direct vision*: Size the Guedel airway by measuring from the middle of the bottom lip to the angle of the jaw. Use a laryngoscope blade as a tongue depressor and light source (or other means of depressing the tongue down and lighting the back of the oropharynx), then pass the Guedel airway over the tongue without any twisting. Airway management can then be continued.

Box 2.2e   Neonatal resuscitation drug dosages – SUMMARY TABLE

Adrenaline; 1:10,000 strength only; 10 mcg/kg (or 0.1 ml/kg), subsequent dosages if necessary. If not effective, increase to..........
30 mcg/kg (0.3 ml/kg) via intravenous route.
Sodium Bicarbonate; 4.2%: 1–2 mmols/kg (2–4 mls/kg)
10% Dextrose; 2–2.5 ml/kg **Volume** (Normal Saline); 10 ml/kg

Reference: Resuscitation Council, 2013

- **Remember ABCD in that order. (Airway, Breathing, Circulation, Drugs). Most newborns require only A and B. Only a few require C and D.**
- **CALL FOR HELP. This is shown throughout the flow chart in Box 2.2a to indicate that there is no set time to call for assistance.**

Resuscitation in the neonatal unit

Resuscitation measures may be necessitated after the period of delivery when neonates are transferred to other areas. Within the special care unit or on the postnatal ward, resuscitation measures may be required in cases where a neonate stops breathing or displays a significant drop in saturations and/or heart rate, with no response to initial intervention, i.e. stimulation and increasing oxygen. Box 2.3 outlines an algorithm for this setting.

Box 2.3   A-B-C Resuscitation in the special care/postnatal unit –
FLOW CHART

Move the neonate to a Resuscitaire® *or* flat, firm surface
Call for help/Access emergency trolley and equipment/Note time
ASSESS ⟹
AIRWAY (Neutral position, suction mouth and/or nose under direct vision *if indicated*) ⟹
▽

BREATHING (use 'T-piece' inflation) or bag-valve mask (BVM) x
5 breaths lasting 2–3 seconds looking for chest movement and/or increase in heart rate ⟹
▽

If no response, re-position airway/provide jaw thrust ⟹
▽

Listen for heart rate and chest movement. If chest is moving and heart rate has increased
▽

Provide ventilation breaths to support breathing
If chest is moving and heart rate is less than 60
▽

CIRCULATION ⟹
▽

Perform cardiac compressions at a ratio of 3:1 (if newborn) OR 15:2 if paediatric guidelines are followed ⟹
▽

Reassess every 30 seconds ⟹
▽

If heart rate remains <60, consider IV access and drugs

🔘 Check local guidance on resuscitation ratio to use after the newborn period as this changes according to age.

✋ The same standard approach highlighted above for the NLS algo-rithm applies to any neonate that requires resuscitation in all settings, again with the main focus on airway and breathing. ▐➡ See also 'Stop and Think' box for Boxes 2.2.

Resuscitation is also required when a ventilated neonate in intensive care suddenly deteriorates; indicated by chest movement ceasing, sudden desaturation, colour change or drop in heart rate. Box 2.4 outlines a flow chart for the intensive care setting.

Box 2.4   Resuscitation in the neonatal intensive care unit – FLOW CHART

ASSESS/Call for medical assistance/Access emergency ventilation ⇒
AIRWAY (Neutral position) ⇒
BREATHING manually ventilate using T-piece or BVM via ETT looking
for chest movement and increase in heart rate. Ventilate at pressures
to achieve chest movement. Listen to air entry
with a stethoscope.

THINK/CONSIDER THE FOLLOWING ...
Displacement of ETT? – is the chest moving both sides? Air entry?

Obstruction of ETT? If chest does not move or no air entry, the ETT may be
blocked. If so, the ETT <u>must</u> be removed and manual ventilation given. Prepare
for reintubation.
▽

Pneumothorax? Unequal chest movement/air entry with a profound
drop in saturation and/or bradycardia? Access the cold light (for
transillumination of the chest) and chest drain equipment if
this is suspected
▽

Pulmonary haemorrhage? Is there frank blood in the ETT?

Equipment malfunction? Are there any ventilation tubing leaks
or equipment faults?
▽

Stiff lungs? The lungs may become less compliant due to collapse, lung
oedema or abdominal distension

Depending on the cause of deterioration, treat/manage as appropriate
▽

⇒ **CIRCULATION** – If heart rate <60 commence cardiac massage

    Check local guidance for resuscitation ratio, as stated in Box 2.3

**Calling for help is vital even when working in the intensive care
setting, no matter how experienced one is. ▐➤ See also 'Stop and
Think' boxes for Boxes 2.2 and 2.3.**

Finally, endotracheal tube (ETT) intubation practice is only necessary if absolutely indicated and when good quality resuscitation by the above measures has not secured the neonate's airway, necessitating ongoing support and insertion of an artificial airway. When this procedure becomes necessary, adequate preparation and guidance are required. Box 2.5 a–c and Table 2.1 include important elements of assisting with intubation in the neonate who requires full ventilation for a given period.

Box 2.5a   Equipment for intubation and endotracheal tube (ETT) fixation – CHECKLIST

- Correct size ETT (see Table 2.1)
- Laryngoscope (check light) with straight blade
- Stethoscope
- Suction with size 8–10 catheter
- T-piece circuit (check pressure) or bag-valve mask (BVM) in working order
- ETT holder and fixation method
- Correct size hat (with ties each side) if used to secure ETT to the holder
- Two pieces of gauze to protect cheeks

Box 2.5b   Nursing responsibilities during intubation – CHECKLIST

- Prepare and assist with administration of sedation and muscle relaxants prior to intubation as prescribed by the medical staff
- Position neonate appropriately for ease of procedure
- Put hat onto neonate first
- While doctor/advanced neonatal nurse practitioner intubates, ensure that suction and bedside resuscitation equipment are available and close to hand
- Observe vital signs and notify person carrying out intubation if oxygen saturation/heart rate drop
- Watch neonate's temperature during exposure ensuring they are kept wrapped and warm
- Once intubation is complete, assist with tube fixation. ETT position can be confirmed by observing chest movement and listening with a stethoscope until an X-ray is obtained (see Box 2.5c)

⦿ Check local guidance for ETT fixation method.

Table 2.1   Guide for ETT sizing – SUMMARY TABLE

Width (2, 2.5, 3, 3.5, 4, 4.5)
General guide <1 kg: 2–2.5/1–2 kg: 2.5–3/2–3 kg: 3–3.5/3–4 kg: 3.5–4/
>4 kg: 4.5

Length to the nearest half centimetre

Corrected gestation (weeks)	Weight (kg)	ETT length at lips (cm)
23–24	0.5–0.6	5.5
25–26	0.7–0.8	6.0
27–29	0.9–1.0	6.5
30–32	1.1–1.4	7.0
33–35	1.5–1.8	7.5
36–37	1.9–2.4	8.0
38–40	2.5–3.1	8.5
41–43	3.2–4.2	9.0

Length is for oral intubation. Add 1 cm for nasal intubation

◉ Check local guidance

Source: Reprinted from Resuscitation, 77 (3), Kempley, S.T., Moreiras, J.W., and Petrone, F.L., Endotracheal tube length for neonatal intubation. Pages 369–373. Copyright (2008), with permission from Elsevier

Box 2.5c   Ascertaining the position of the ETT– CHECKLIST

- **Clinical assessment**: chest movement and air entry should be present and equal on both sides
- **Chest X-ray (CXR)** for confirmation of ETT position after insertion to above lengths. The tube length should then be adjusted from the original insertion position to align the tip with the thoracic vertebrae T1—T2 (Kempley et al., 2008)
- ETT tip should be between 0.2 cm and 2 cm above the carina (Schmölzer et al., 2013)
- The most common incorrect positioning is in the right mainstem bronchus
- **Calorimetric end tidal carbon dioxide (EtCO$_2$) detector** can be used prior to CXR (Harigopal and Satish, 2008) – e.g. the 'Pedicap', a disposable

(continued)

ETT connection containing a pH sensitive indicator. If carbon dioxide (CO_2) is detected in the expired breaths, this is an indication that the ETT is in the correct position. An absence of colour change suggests that the tube is not in the trachea (Schmölzer et al., 2013)

◉ Check local guidance on methods of ETT sizing, ascertaining position and fixation

---

🖐️ **Close observation is a vital nursing role during the intubation procedure to support whoever is carrying this out, particularly of the heart rate and oxygen saturation levels.**

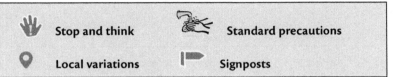

🖐️ **Stop and think**   ✋ **Standard precautions**

◉ **Local variations**   ▶ **Signposts**

✋ **Always apply standard precautions. Wash hands and wear gloves and aprons during procedures such as resuscitation and intubation.**

◉ **The space below can be used to record any local variations and practice points specific to your own unit.**

Airway: Glossary

Airway: The passage by which air enters the lungs for ventilation. Without a patent airway, breathing and circulation will cease.

Bag-valve mask (BVM): A self-inflating bag which is a hand-held device, used to provide positive pressure ventilation to neonates who are not breathing adequately.

Breathing: The process of inhaling and exhaling air in and out of the lungs for gaseous exchange. Also known as 'ventilation'.

Circulation: The movement of blood around the body as a result of the heart's pumping action.

Cold light: Fibre-optic light used to transilluminate the chest wall.

Endotracheal tube (ETT): Small plastic tube that is inserted through a neonate's nose or mouth down through the larynx and into the trachea for full mechanical ventilation.

Intubation: Insertion of an ETT into the trachea when full ventilation support is required (extubation is the removal of the ETT).

Laryngoscope: An instrument for examining the larynx, or for inserting an ETT through it.

PEEP valve: A dial on the end of a ventilator circuit, which sets and maintains positive end expiratory pressure (PEEP) at the end of exhalation by means of mechanical impedance.

Resuscitaire®: A portable overhead radiant heater providing a flat surface and a means of delivering gases and pressure via a ventilation circuit to a neonate who requires resuscitation.

T-piece: A ventilation circuit attached to a gas source used for manual ventilation by occluding the top of the T-shaped connector attached to the ETT.

⏩ The Glossary for *Assessment* is also relevant for this topic and can be referred to for terminology relating to assessment during resuscitation and thereafter. Glossaries for *Breathing* and *Oxygen therapy* also contain related terms.

Airway: References

Atkinson, E., Summers, D., Jones H., and Barrington, J. (2010). Neonatal resuscitation – A practical approach. The experience of one UK tertiary neonatal unit. *Infant.* 6 (1): 9–14.

Harigopal, S., and Satish, H.P. (2008). End-tidal carbon dioxide monitoring in neonates. *Infant.* 4 (2): 51–53.

Kempley, S.T., Moreiras, J.W., and Petrone, F.L. (2008). Endotracheal tube length for neonatal intubation. *Resuscitation.* 77: 369–373.

Ramji, S., Rasaily, R., Mishra, P.K., Narang, A., Jayam, S., Kapoor, A.N., et al. (2003). Resuscitation of asphyxiated newborns with room air or 100% oxygen at birth: A multicentre clinical trial. *Indian Pediatr.* 40 (5): 10–517.

Resuscitation Council (2013). *Newborn Life Support Manual (3rd edition).* Resuscitation Council, London www.resus.org.uk/.

Schmölzer, G.M., O'Reilly, M., Davis, P.G., Cheung, P.Y., and Roehr, C.C. (2013). Confirmation of correct tracheal tube placement in newborn infants. *Resuscitation.* 84 (6): 731–737.

Tan, A., Schulze, A., O'Donnell, C., and Davis, P. (2005). Air versus oxygen for resuscitation of infants at birth. *Cochrane Database Systematic Rev.* (2): CD002273.

Assessment

Assessment is an essential nursing skill that forms the basis of any decision and subsequent intervention. As seen in the previous unit, it is an integral and vital component of resuscitation at the beginning, during the actual process and following the stabilization and subsequent care of a neonate requiring airway management. It is important to ascertain and understand what the normal assessment criteria are, so that any deviations from this can be noted and appropriate intervention undertaken. Assessment should be individualized to the specific neonate and situation or condition, holistically considering all systems, including the family and psychosocial needs. This section focuses on various clinical assessment tools (Tables 2.2–2.8c, Boxes 2.6–2.8, and Figure 2.3) from the period of birth and into ongoing neonatal care including screening (Table 2.2 and Box 2.4).

Related topics: Assessment is a vital component of *any* aspect of care within this book. For example, see *Airway, Breathing* and *Cardiovascular care* since assessment is an integral thread throughout the A-B-C approach. It is also essential for any other care practice such as assessing for *infection, jaundice* and *skin care*.

Table 2.2	Assessment of the newborn at delivery – SUMMARY TABLE
Heart rate	• Heart rate should be ideally greater than 100bpm, if well at birth. • It may be absent or less than 100 in a compromised newborn at birth.
Respiratory effort	• There should be good respiratory effort at birth. A crying newborn indicates the airway is open. • A compromised newborn may be gasping or display difficulties breathing and if they are very hypoxic, breathing may be absent.
Muscle tone	• A healthy newborn will display good muscle tone and limb flexion. • A compromised newborn may show reduced tone or appear floppy
Response to stimulation	• A good response to stimulation at birth would be a cry and spontaneous, vigorous movement. • A compromised newborn will show a slow or no response.
Colour	• A healthy newborn, although may appear peripherally blue in colour initially, should be centrally pink. Hands and feet should start to show as pink within the first hour of life (watch specifically the mucous membranes, lips and nail beds to accommodate all skin tones). • A compromised newborn will appear white (pallor) or blue centrally (cyanosis)

(continued)

Table 2.2   Continued
Considering these areas with other information in Box 2.6 will determine subsequent management.

Note: If a traditional 'Apgar' score is assigned (Apgar, 1953), a score of 0, 1 or 2 is given for the each of the above areas. 0 indicates an absent or poor response. 1 is when there is some response but this is insufficient or of concern. 2 is given where there is a good response in a healthy newborn. The scores are totalled to ascertain a score between 0–10 taken at 1, 5 and 10 minutes of age.

 Observe local guidance on the agreed system used to assess the newborn baby.

Box 2.6   Additional information for assessment at birth –CHECKLIST

To ascertain the presence of fetal compromise if available. Consider:
Blood gas analysis of cord blood, preferably both arterial and venous
Monitoring data during labour or presence of thick meconium

Cord care at birth:

If the newborn is 'well', delay cord clamping for 1 minute and give to parents for skin-to-skin holding.
If requiring intervention for concern, immediate cord clamping is performed
▐➡ See Umbilical care chapter, and newborn life support (NLS) flow chart commenced (see Box 2.2a).

Antenatal history. Ask:

• Were there any pregnancy complications?

Perinatal factors. Ask:

• Fetal and/or cord blood gas, cardiotocography (CTG) monitoring, fetal compromise?
• What was the method of delivery?
• What is the gestation of the neonate? Was this preterm labour?
• Has mother received antenatal steroids during preterm labour?

Assessment at birth. Ask:

• Was there a need to employ the NLS flow chart? ▐➡ See Box 2.2a–e.
• Were the following criteria satisfactory at birth: response to stimulation, colour, tone, heart rate and breathing? ▐➡ See Table 2.2
• Ensure Vitamin K is administered by appropriate route, according to national and local guidance.
• Is the neonate preterm, so necessitating specific early care? ▐➡ See Figure 2.3 and Table 2.4–2.5.

 Check local guidance

> ✋ The 5 components that make up the traditional 'Apgar score' (Apgar, 1953) give practitioners a picture of whether resuscitation interventions are required or if there is a cause for any concern, even if a formal score is not assigned.

Assessment after delivery

A neonate who requires admission to the neonatal unit (NNU) following compromise before, during or after birth will require a full assessment, which should be documented carefully in order to ascertain baseline values, as well as guide subsequent interventions. Table 2.3 and Box 2.7 outline summary guides for areas of assessment to cover on admission and thereafter.

Table 2.3   Clinical assessment of the neonate – SUMMARY TABLE

☛ For 'normal' ranges and parameters for vital signs, refer to Box 2.8.

System	Normal/expected assessment criteria	Assessment criteria indicating compromise and requiring action
Airway and breathing (respiratory)	Self-ventilating neonate Effortless breathing which may be periodic, normal rate, bilateral chest movement, pink in colour, quiet chest sounds, no oxygen requirement, oxygen saturations within normal range. Ventilated neonate Even, bilateral chest movement, air entry clear and bilateral, no secretions evident, ETT fixed and secure. Minimum oxygen requirement.	Tachypnoea, nasal flaring, chest recession, apnoea, oxygen requirement, grunting, cyanosis, abnormal chest sounds; e.g. stridor/wheeze, oxygen requirement, poor oxygen saturations. Absent or uneven chest movement, excess secretions, absent breath sounds on one or both sides.
Cardiovascular	Adequate mean blood pressure (MBP), capillary refill less than 3 seconds, urine output at least 1 ml/kg/hour, mucous membranes pink in colour, warm skin, palpable pulses, and heart rate within normal limits.	MBP below desired limit, pale, cool skin, low/diminishing urine output, capillary refill >3 seconds, weak and thready pulses, tachycardia initially, then bradycardia (late sign).

(continued)

Table 2.3   Continued

System	Normal/expected assessment criteria	Assessment criteria indicating compromise and requiring action
Developmental/ behavioural and stress	No presence of pain or stress. Neonate is positioned appropriately-flexed, limbs in mid-line, appears comfortable, relaxed and able to sleep for long periods.	Presence of pain or stress cues: tense, continual movements, facial expressions, excessive crying and grimace, changes to vital signs, colour change, apnoea and desaturations.
Environmental/ thermal control	Normal body temperature (36.5–37.2 degrees Celsius) and appropriate environmental temperature according to age, gestation and birth weight.	Temperature <36.5 or >37.2 degrees Celsius – i.e. thermal instability (or 'thermal stress') is present.
Fluid status and balance	Adequate systemic perfusion and urine output, normal fontanelles, palpable peripheral pulses, good skin turgor, normal sodium level, specific gravity of urine 1.010–1.020, weight gain appropriate for age, adequate fluid balance.	Fluid depleted – Low urine output (<1 ml/kg/ hour) (see above), sunken fontanelles, dry skin, fast and thready pulses, high specific gravity, large decreases in weight, large negative fluid balance. Fluid overload - Polyuria, bulging fontanelles, low specific gravity, large increases in weight, positive fluid balance.
Gastro-intestinal and nutritional status	Soft, non-tender abdomen, bowel sounds, nil/minimal aspirate from stomach which is clear and mucousy, bowels open and normal stool, no vomiting, tolerance of feeds if applicable.	Distended, tender, hard abdomen, no bowel sounds or bowel actions, stool bloody/too loose/ green/large and/or increasing stomach aspirates, bile aspirates, vomiting, failure to tolerate feeds.
The three Hs (metabolic adaptation)	Able to maintain adequate oxygenation, body temperature and blood glucose. Oxygenation and body temperature – see above, blood glucose, >2.6 mmols in first few hours, then 4–6 mmols thereafter.	Failure of normal metabolic adaptation leading to the three Hs – hypoxia, hypothermia and hypoglycaemia (<2.6 mmol/l). Hyperglycaemia >8 mmol/l.

(continued)

Table 2.3   Continued

System	Normal/expected assessment criteria	Assessment criteria indicating compromise and requiring action
Immunological	Signs of infection are not evident.	Signs of infection may be non-specific and include respiratory distress, colour change, low oxygen saturation, increasing oxygen requirement, changes in vital signs, apnoea.
Jaundice (hepatic)	Physiological jaundice due to liver immaturity is common: noted by yellow skin on blanching and yellow sclera of eyes. Serum or transcutaneous bilirubin below treatment threshold.	Jaundice that exceeds threshold bilirubin level requiring treatment or *pathological* jaundice – early onset and due to a disease process.
Musculoskeletal	Presence of well-toned and flexed posture with spontaneous movements.	Abnormal posture and tone, e.g. hypo- or hypertonia.
Neurological and sensory	Response to stimuli is present. Neonate is alert, wakes for feeds and is able to feed. Normal/present reflexes are exhibited commensurate with gestation and age.	Unresponsive or less responsive to stimuli, excessive wakefulness or poor levels of consciousness, changes in behaviour. Abnormal movements such as convulsions.
Skin and general appearance	Normal skin for gestation, e.g. frail and red in the preterm, and well formed in term, pink mucous membranes, no excoriation, no signs of jaundice, umbilical area clean, intravenous (IV) sites healthy.	Broken, excoriated skin, rashes and tissued IV sites or suspected clinical jaundice, blue mucous membranes.

🔘 Check local guidance for required assessment information

References: Lomax (2011); Petty (2011); Hazinski (2012); Rennie and Kendal (2013)

The focus of the above guide is physical assessment. However, family adjustment to admission to a neonatal unit, along with their psychosocial needs must also be considered as part of the holistic assessment of the neonate and family. ▶ This will be covered in detail in *Psychosocial care of the family*.

🖐 **While assessment as applied to the *systems* can help impart a systematic structure to the process, it should be considered within a holistic perspective. For example, any vital sign must be interpreted** according to the individual neonate's condition alongside clinical assessment and, if applicable, blood values. ▰▶ See *Blood*.

Box 2.7   Assessment on admission to the neonatal unit – CHECKLIST

Area of assessment	Examples of what to consider A systematic approach to assessment includes ABC and beyond
A	• **A**irway – is it open and patent? What airway support is required?
	• **A**ssessment – vital sign observations/monitoring – heart rate, respiratory status, blood pressure, oxygen saturation, blood gas analysis values, blood glucose, admission screen/swabs
	• **B**reathing – does the neonate require respiratory support?
	• **C**irculation – do they require cardiovascular support?
	• **D**rugs – do they require any specific drug therapy?
	• **E**nvironment – is the environment prepared and conducive to their needs?
	• **F**luid requirement – what fluid regime are they on?
	• **G**astrointestinal/bowels – passed meconium? Abdomen?
	• **H-** The three Hs (hypoxia, hypoglycaemia or hypothermia)?
	• **I**nfection – are there any signs of actual or risk of sepsis?
	• **J**aundice – what is the serum bilirubin? Clinical jaundice?
	• **K-** Vitamin K – has this been administered?/Kangaroo care – applicable?
	• **L**evel of dependency
	• **M**ulti-disciplinary team (MDT) involvement – consider referrals
	• **N**eurological signs present?
	• **O**xygen requirement and monitoring?
	• **P**arents, family care and psychosocial needs?
	• **Q**uality, risk and safeguarding – always be mindful at the outset
	• **R**enal/urine – passed urine? Output?
	• **S**urgical neonate/skin integrity
	• **T**ransfer required? Temperature and thermal control?
	• **U**mbilical lines – are these necessary?
	• **V**omiting?
	• **W**eight?
X	• **X**-rays – what are required as part of the assessment above?
	▰▶ There are chapters for all of the above points which cover these topics in more detail

 Check local guidance for specific admission documentation

> ✋ **Assessment of a 'baseline' is essential for any neonatal admission and is the starting point for any interventions. All admission assessments must be documented. |➡ See Box 2.20**

Assessment of the preterm neonate

The neonatal unit (NNU) admits a significant number of preterm neonates for varying levels of care and intervention, many of which are classed as *extremely preterm*. Optimum stabilization in the early hours of life of these very vulnerable neonates is of the utmost importance to optimize their outcome (Chalmers and Mears, 2005) and there are some specific assessment factors for this group of neonates that require emphasis. Table 2.4 outlines specific differences relevant to the preterm neonate for clinical assessment and Table 2.5 depicts some key clinical features that can be used to ascertain a neonate's gestational age if this is unknown. Assessment and stabilization of the preterm neonate at birth, a term known as the 'Golden Hour' (Doyle and Bradshaw, 2012), is outlined in Figure 2.3, which applies to the preterm neonate at less than 32 weeks gestation. However, a distinction is made between two further sub-sets within this group: those born at less than 28 weeks gestation and those born *between* 28 weeks and up to 32 weeks.

> |➡ There are many integral topics relevant to the care of the preterm neonate throughout this book: See particularly *Developmental care, Environmental care, The three Hs, Respiratory distress, Thermal care* and *Weight.*

Table 2.4   Clinical assessment of the preterm neonate – SUMMARY TABLE

System	*Compared to the term neonate,* the *key* specific features of the preterm neonate are ....
Airway and breathing (respiratory)	Immature lung function and surfactant deficiency. Alveoli are more fragile and easily damaged. Underdeveloped respiratory centre (brain stem) leads to a predisposition to apnoea of prematurity.
Cardiovascular	Less efficient cardiac output due to immaturity of the heart muscle and reduced contractility. Total blood volume is reduced. Higher acceptable heart rate and lower limits for mean blood pressure (MBP).

(continued)

Table 2.4   Continued

Developmental/ behavioural/stress	Not able to display the same behavioural states, posture or movement shown at term due to immaturity and lack of muscle development, tone, strength and inability to cry. May exhibit different stress signs or cues.
Environmental/ thermal control	Increased risk of hypothermia due to lack of brown and subcutaneous fat, increased surface area to volume ratio. More vulnerable to environmental stressors within the extra-uterine environment.
Fluid status and balance	Immature kidneys that are not able to tolerate large volumes and can easily become overloaded.
Gastro-intestinal and nutrition	Immature gut function and inability to feed orally due to underdeveloped suck-swallow reflexes.
The three Hs – metabolic adaptation	Limited glycogen stores and nutritional reserves laid down normally in pregnancy that are more easily exhausted in response to compromise. The preterm neonate is less able to achieve normal metabolic adaptation to extra-uterine life.
Immunological	Prematurity means that neonates will fail to receive the transfer of immunoglobulins across the placenta that normally occurs during the last trimester of pregnancy and they will consequently be immunocompromised.
Jaundice (hepatic)	Physiological jaundice is more common due to liver immaturity. Lowered threshold for treatment of jaundice.
Musculoskeletal	Poor muscular tone before 34 weeks gestation.
Neurological and sensory	Immature germinal matrix (vascular) layer of the brain ventricles under 34 weeks; more prone to intra-ventricular haemorrhage (IVH).
Skin and general appearance	Underdeveloped and poorly waterproofed skin due to lack of keratin.

References: Petty (2011); Rennie and Kendal (2013)

The preterm neonate is physiologically immature in all of the above systems, making them particularly vulnerable to the effects of the extra-uterine environment and the impact of neonatal care practices.

Figure 2.3 Stabilization of the preterm neonate:
the 'Golden Hour' – FLOW CHART

• AT BIRTH

• **All (<32 weeks)** : assess need for airway management/NLS algorithm (see *Airway*). Use pulse oximetry to ascertain oxygen requirement (see *Oxygen administration*)

• **28–32 weeks**: as above *if stable/well*, delay cord clamping, wrap and keep warm, apply skin-to-skin as appropriate

• **<28 weeks or unstable neonate 28–32 weeks requiring support**: immediate cord clamping, place neonate in plastic bag (<28–30 weeks) under radiant heater, dry head and put on hat, give airway and breathing support as gently as possible, limit inflation breath pressures

• FIRST HOUR

• **All (<32 weeks)**: key areas are stabilization of airway and breathing, close assessment, sound thermal care, prevention of hypothermia, hypoglycaemia and hypoxia (*The three Hs*)

• **28–32 weeks**: as above. Low threshold for intubation and ventilation. Limit oxygen as much as possible; use pulse oximetry and apply limits (see Table 2.29)

• **<28 weeks**: early surfactant is recommended and the subsequent use of CPAP as tolerated to avoid ventilation. Give oxygen with caution and apply limits as above. Leave neonate in plastic bag and remove bag when inside humidified incubator (up to 85% humidity). (See *Thermal care*). Give gentle handling. (See *Developmental care*) ☞

• SUBSEQUENT CARE

• **All preterm neonates (<32 weeks)**: aim for early extubation if ventilated, use of CPAP, continued thermal control and humidification, gentle handling and avoidance of stress and pain –no routine suction, minimize environmental influences, early nutrition.

• **For all**: the birth of a preterm neonate has a significant emotional impact on parents. Ensure their needs and anxieties are considered within the 'Golden Hour' and thereafter (Doyle and Bradshaw, 2012). (See *Psychosocial* care of the family).

⚲ Check local guidance for specific information on care of the preterm neonate

✋ What happens in the 'Golden Hour' can influence the later outcome of an extremely preterm neonate (Bissinger and Annibale, 2010; Castrodale and Rinehart, 2014).

Table 2.5 Assessment of gestational age – SUMMARY TABLE

SIGN	Extreme preterm ⟶			Mid-trimester ⟶		Term ⟶	Post-term
Skin	Sticky, friable, transparent	Gelatinous, red, translucent	Smooth pink, visible veins	Fewer visible veins	Intact skin, pink, rare veins	Fully formed intact skin at term, no vessels	Leathery, cracked, wrinkled
Lanugo hair	None	Sparse	Ample	Thinning	Bald areas	Mostly bald	As for term
Creases of foot (plantar surface)	No creases	No creases	Faint red marks	Anterior transverse creases only	2/3 creases	Creases over entire sole	As for term
Breast	Not obvious	Barely perceptible	Flat, no bud	Small bud	Raised areola	Full areola	As for term
Eye/ear	Lids fused	Lids open Ear pinna flat and soft	Curved pinna but soft	Well curved pinna with good recoil	Formed and firm	Thick ear cartilage	As for term
Genitals (male)	Flat smooth scrotum	Scrotum empty	Testes in upper canal	Testes descending, few rugae	Testes down, good rugae	Descended with deep rugae	As for term
Genitals (female)	Clitoris prominent and labia flat	As previous but small labia minora	As previous growing labia minora	Majora and minora equally prominent	Labia majora large and minora small	Labia majora covers minora	As for term
Posture		Flat and extended	Mild tone present	Some flexion, upper limbs more so than lower	Improved tone and flexion of all limbs	All limbs flexed and toned	As for term

⬛ See also *Weight* which includes a guide to distinguishing between growth restricted and preterm neonates.

Source: Adapted from J Pediatr, 119 (3), Ballard J.L. Khoury, J.C, Wedig, K, Wang, L, Eilers-Walsman, B.L. & Lipp. R. New Ballard Score, expanded to include extremely premature infants. Pages 417–423. Copyright (1991), with permission from Elsevier and Dr. J. Ballard

> ✋ **Knowing the gestational age in weeks of a neonate on admission is important to guide appropriate management.**

Taking observations

Taking observations of key vital signs is a fundamental nursing skill. It is important that norms specific to the neonate are understood so that any deviation from these norms is quickly identified. Tables 2.6–2.7 and Box 2.8 outline the methods used to take vital signs, the normal parameters and the principles of setting appropriate alarm limits.

Table 2.6   Taking vital signs in the neonate – SUMMARY TABLE

Interval	Continuous
Body temperature	
Up to 1 month old: axilla by digital thermometer **Over 1 month old:** axilla by chemical thermometer, leave for 3 minutes with the dots against the neonate's trunk and read 10 seconds after removal, OR axilla by digital thermometer (as above) OR tympanic thermometer placed in ear canal (NICE, 2013; RCN, 2013)	Abdominal or axilla readings can be taken continuously by a probe which reads and displays the temperature. This can be set to influence the heat delivered by the incubator or overhead heater ('Servo' control). Alternatively, the latter can be set manually ('Manual' control). (➡ See *Thermal care*) In addition, a probe on the foot allows peripheral temperature to be observed to consider the core-toe temperature gap
Heart rate	
Apex – place bell of the stethoscope on the apex area, usually to the left of the sternum, between the nipples. Record beats/minute	Electrocardiograph (ECG). Ensure good sinus rhythm is visible on the monitor
Pulse	
The brachial or femoral pulse can be palpated in the neonate (under 1 year of age)	Continuous pulse can be monitored via a pulse oximeter (see overleaf)
Blood pressure	
Non-invasive (cuff) – ensure the cuff covers most of the length of the upper arm or lower leg and circles 90–100% of the circumference. Straighten the limb and keep it still during reading. Either use 'manual' or set the monitor to 'automatic' to record at regular intervals	Invasive (arterial) blood pressure – ensure the set-up has been calibrated (zeroed) and the transducer is at the level of the heart. Ensure a good trace and optimize. Record hourly. (➡ See *Box 2.19 a and b in Cardiovascular system care*)

(continued)

Table 2.6   Continued

Respiratory rate

Observe the chest and count/record breaths per minute. Look for even chest movement, bilateral, ease of breathing	ECG leads will read a continuous respiratory trace. This should also be checked manually at intervals

Oxygen saturation

Continuous only: A saturation probe attached to a pulse oximeter is placed around a pulsatile area – e.g. foot, hand, wrist and the O_2 saturation (SpO_2) and pulse are continuously measured.
(☞ See *Tables 2.28 and 2.29 in Oxygen therapy*)

Transcutaneous oxygen

Continuous only: A probe is calibrated every 2–4 hours and then placed on a flat surface of skin – e.g. chest. (☞ As above)

End tidal carbon dioxide (EtCO$_2$)

Continuous only: CO_2 in exhaled breath is measured at the end of expiration by chemical reaction (calorimetry), or by measuring molecules providing a numerical value (capnometer)

Capillary refill time (CRT)

Blanch skin for 5 seconds and count how many seconds for colour (perfusion) to return

Urine output

Divide urine (ml) passed in a given time period by the weight and by the number of hours

○ Check local guidance on devices used for taking vital signs in conjunction with company guidelines

---

🖐 **All vital signs should be recorded clearly and accurately every hour if a neonate is on continuous monitoring or at intervals, varying from 1–4 hours. After continuous monitoring has ceased, frequency of vital sign taking and recording generally depends on the individual patient and agreed accordingly (RCN, 2013).**

Box 2.8   A Guide to neonatal parameters and values – CHECKLIST

Heart rate; beats per minute (bpm)		
Age	Awake	Sleeping
Neonate (preterm)	100–200	120–180
Neonate (term)	100–180	80–160
Infant	100–160	75–160
Toddler	80–110	60–90
Pre-schooler	70–110	60–90
School	65–110	60–90
Blood pressure (mmHg)		
Age	Systolic	Diastolic
Birth (12 hr, <1 kg)	39–59	16–36
Birth (12 hr, 3 kg)	50–70	24–45
Neonate (96 hr)	60–90	20–60
Infant (6 month)	87–105	53–66
Toddler (2 year)	95–105	53–66
School age	97–112	57–71
Adult	112–128	66–80

N.B: In the neonatal unit, it is vital to consider the **mean arterial blood pressure**.
As a *general* guide, the gestational age in weeks should correspond with mean BP.
(☞ See *Cardiovascular system care*)

Respiratory rates: breaths per minute (bpm)	
Preterm	40–80 bpm
Term neonates	30–70
Infants	30–60
Toddlers	24–40
Preschool	22–34
School/adult	18–30

(continued)

Temperature	
Central (axilla)	36.6–37.2 degrees Celsius
Abdominal (probe)	36.6–37.2 (preterm) 35.5–36.5 degrees (term)
Peripheral (foot)	34.6–36.2
Core-toe temperature gap	less than 2 degrees Celsius

Oxygen monitoring ➤ See *Tables 2.28 and 2.29 in Oxygen therapy*

Perfusion	
Capillary refill time (CRT)	less than 3 seconds (RCN, 2013)
Urine output	minimum of 1 ml/kg hour

Circulating blood volume	
Neonates	85–90 ml/kg
Infants	75–80
Children	70–75
Adults	65–70

Tidal volumes	
Neonates	4–6 ml/kg
Children	6–10 ml/kg

Glucose
>2.6 mmol in the at-risk/sick neonate ➤ See Box 2.14 in Blood
4–6 mmol after the newborn period and in children/adults

📍 Check local guidance on parameters

References: Hazinski, 2012; Rennie and Kendall, 2013

🖐 **Understanding a normal range is important to serve as a baseline with which to compare assessed parameters and whether these require attention. All values are <u>averages</u> and should serve as a guideline.**

Table 2.7   Setting alarm limits: general principles – SUMMARY TABLE

Vital sign	Setting limits
Heart rate	100–200 bpm
Respiratory rate	30–80 breaths per min
Mean blood pressure (MBP)	Consider gestational age in weeks for acceptable norm of MBP ☞ See Box 2.8 and Box 2.19a in *Cardiovascular system care* For sick preterm neonate, keep MBP above 30 mmHg For sick term neonate, keep MBP above 40 mmHg This needs to be discussed at local unit level according to the individual condition of the specific neonate ♀
Oxygen saturations	Any neonate in air 90–100% Term hypoxic neonate 95–100% Preterm: SpO_2 should be targeted at 90–95% until the infant reaches 36 weeks' postconceptual age. (Stenson et al, 2011; Saugstad and Aune, 2014) ☞ See Table 2.29 in *Oxygen therapy*
Transcutaneous oxygen and CO_2	Aim for the same limits as for blood gas values PaO_2 6.5–10 kPa (preterm)/6.5–12 kPa (infant/child) $PaCO_2$ 4–6 kPa

⚲ Check local guidance on agreed/accepted ranges, values and upper/lower limits

✋ **Setting upper and lower acceptable limits should be done according to the neonate's age, gestation and condition taking into account factors such as sleep/wake states, activity and stress levels.**

Screening in the neonate

Screening is an important area of healthcare and is necessary for the early identification of risks for certain diseases in order to take timely action following a diagnosis as appropriate. Antenatal screening may have identified neonates at risk even prior to delivery.

Tables 2.8a–d provide an overview to guide four main areas of screening in the neonatal period; bloodspot screening, retinopathy of prematurity, hearing and examination of the newborn, respectively. Appropriate recommendations are made by the NHS National Screening Committee http://newbornphysical.screening.nhs.uk for all areas of screening including both antenatal and postnatal tests.

🖐 **Screening identifies a risk of having or developing a disease. It is *not* a diagnosis.**

Table 2.8   Screening overview – SUMMARY TABLE

HOW?	WHY?

Table 2.8a   Bloodspot screening in the neonatal unit

o Within 5 days of birth, a single blood spot is saved to send with the 5–8 day test. o Day 5, full blood spot test (unless a blood transfusion has been given). o If a blood transfusion has been given, wait 72 hours before taking the full blood spot test (no later than day 8). o In neonates born <36 weeks, repeat single blood spot at 28 days. o Record all tests in medical notes – indicate date, whether a repeat test and sign. o When multiple blood transfusions and no pre-transfusion blood spot was taken, a repeat test is arranged at 3 months after last transfusion.	Eight autosomal, recessive genetic disorders are screened for: • Phenylketonuria (PKU) • Sickle cell disease • Medium chain acyl coenzyme A dehydrogenase deficiency (MCADD) • Cystic fibrosis (CF) • Maple syrup urine disease (MSUD) • Isovaleric acidaemia (IVA) • Glutaric aciduria type 1 (GA1) • Homocystinuria (HCU) In addition, • Congenital hypothyroidism • Surveillance for maternal human immunodeficiency virus (HIV) (anonymous testing, not individual diagnosis). Metabolic disorders such as PKU and congenital hypothyroidism are conditions, which, if untreated, can result in significant developmental delay.
For full information on national guidance, see http://newbornscreening-bloodspot.org.uk	

🖐 **All screening should be explained to the parents including reasons for performing it and actions if required.**

Table 2.8b   Retinopathy of prematurity

How?	Why?
Retinopathy of prematurity (ROP) screening is undertaken for: o All neonates with a birth weight of less than 1500 g	Done to detect, identify stage and treat ROP as appropriate, as follows:

(continued)

Table 2.8b   Continued

How?	Why?
o All neonates 31 weeks or less o 1st examination is taken at 6–7 weeks postnatal age or post-conceptual age of 36 weeks o Prior to examination cyclopentolate 0.5% and phenylephrine 2.5% eye drops are prescribed and administered prior to arrival of ophthalmologist o Repeat every 2 weeks or according to individual assessment by ROP team o **Location of ROP** – Each zone (1–3) is centred in relation to the optic disc as the focal point o **Extent of ROP** – Recorded as clock hours	**Stage 1: Demarcation line** – thin flat line separating the vascular and avascular retina **Stage 2: Ridge** – the ridge extends above the retina **Stage 3: Proliferation** of blood vessels (neovascularization) extends from the ridge into the vitreous fluid **Stage 4: Partial retinal detachment** **Stage 5: Total retinal detachment**

⬤ In line with national guidance (RCPCH/RCO/BAPM, 2008), also observe local guidance on ROP screening

References: International Committee for the Classification of Retinopathy of Prematurity (2005); RCPCH/RCO/BAPM (2008)

✋ Determination of the stage, location and extent of ROP is used to decide on the need for later treatment by laser or cryotherapy.

Table 2.8c   Neonatal hearing screening

How?	Why?
• ALL neonates should have hearing screening prior to discharge OR arranged for community follow-up before 6 weeks (post-term corrected age). • The screen uses two tests called the Otoacoustic emissions (OAEs) test and the Automated Auditory Brainstem Response test (AABR). Both tests are painless.	The aim is to identify any hearing loss that could go on to affect language acquisition in the developing infant/child. In turn, intervention is given as soon as possible to prevent a delay in this vital area of development. Neonates who do not show strong responses will be referred for a full diagnostic assessment.

Full information and national guidance, see http://www.nhsp.info/

✋ The implications of hearing loss in the at-risk neonate must be considered in line with consideration of future sensory outcomes.

Table 2.8d Physical examination of the neonate	
When?	**Why?**
Ideally, physical examination should take place: • At birth • Within the first 24 hours • At 72 hours • At 6 weeks	To detect any condition, anomaly or dysmorphic feature that may need early treatment and referral.

How? A full examination should include:

- a review of the health history of the family, mother and neonate
- head (including fontanelles), face, nose, mouth including palate, ears, neck and general symmetry of head and facial features. Note head circumference
- eyes; check opacities and 'red reflex'
- neck and clavicles, limbs, hands, feet and digits; assess proportions and symmetry
- heart; check position, rate, rhythm and sounds, murmurs and femoral pulse volume
- lungs; check effort, rate and sounds
- abdomen; check shape and palpate to identify any organomegaly, umbilical cord
- genitalia and anus; check for completeness and patency and undescended testes in males
- spine; palpate bony structures and check integrity of skin
- skin; note colour and texture as well as birthmarks or rashes
- central nervous system; check tone, behaviour, movements and posture and reflexes
- hips; check symmetry of limbs and skin folds
- cry; note sound
- weight

References: NHS National Screening Committee (2015) and Lomax (2011)

 Full guidance should be referred to for any screening. The above offers a summary and short synopsis only.

 Stop and think   **Standard precautions**

 Local variations   **Signposts**

Always apply standard precautions. Wash hands thoroughly before and after handling neonates during assessment.

The space below can be used to record any local variations and practice points specific to your own unit.

Assessment: glossary

Anomaly: Deviation from what is standard, normal or expected (see *Congenital*).

Apgar score: An assessment score ranging from 0 to 10 indicating a newborn's physical condition immediately following birth. Developed by Virginia Apgar in 1953 ©.

Automated Auditory Brainstem Response (AABR) test: One of two hearing screening tests. A stimulus is presented using earphones or probe and the electrophysiological response from the brainstem is detected by electrodes placed on the scalp.

Blood spot screening: The term used to describe the mandatory newborn screening carried out via heel prick from day 5 of life. The conditions screened for are:

Congenital hypothyroidism (CH): A condition of thyroid hormone deficiency which can arise as a problem with thyroid gland development or of genetic origin.

Cystic fibrosis (CF): A disorder which affects the exocrine glands and the body's ability to move salt and water in and out of cells causing the lungs and pancreas to secrete abnormally thick mucus that can block the airway and prevent proper functioning.

Glutaric aciduria type 1 (GA1): An inherited disorder in which the body is unable to break down the amino acids lysine, hydroxylysine and tryptophan.

Homocystinuria (HCU): A disorder of methionine metabolism, leading to an abnormal accumulation of homocysteine and its metabolites in blood and urine.

Human immunodeficiency virus (HIV): See *Infection*.

Isovaleric acidaemia (IVA): Or isovaleric acid CoA dehydrogenase deficiency, is a rare autosomal recessive metabolic disorder which disrupts or prevents normal metabolism of the amino acid leucine. It is a type of organic academia.

Maple syrup urine disease (MSUD): An autosomal recessive metabolic disorder affecting branched-chain amino acids. It is one type of organic acidemia. The condition gets its name from the distinctive sweet odour of urine.

Medium chain acyl coenzyme A dehydrogenase deficiency (MCADD): A disorder that results from the lack of an enzyme required to metabolize fat into energy.

Phenylketonuria (PKU): An autosomal recessive genetic disorder detected by high levels of phenylalanine in the blood which, if not detected and treated, causes metabolites to accumulate resulting in brain damage.

Sickle cell disease: A haemoglobinopathy that affects the normal oxygen carrying capacity of red blood cells due to abnormal, sickle-cell shaped haemoglobin. Beta thalassaemia is another haemoglobinopathy.

Bradycardia: Slow heart rate.

Capnography: Monitoring of the concentration of carbon dioxide in the respiratory gases.

Cardiopulmonary monitor: A machine that monitors a neonate's heart and breathing rates connected by adhesive pads placed on the chest, which displays information on a screen.

Cardiotocography (CTG): A means of recording the fetal heartbeat and the uterine contractions during labour.

Congenital: Relating to a condition that develops before and is present at birth. For example, a congenital anomaly can also be termed 'birth defect'.

Cryotherapy: Freezing of abnormal tissue to halt its growth. Used in severe cases of retinopathy of prematurity although laser treatment is more commonly used.

Cyanosis: A blue discolouration of the skin caused by insufficient oxygen.

Dysmorphic feature: A medical term referring to a difference of body structure that can be an isolated feature or it can be suggestive of a congenital disorder, genetic syndrome, or birth defect.

End tidal carbon dioxide monitoring (EtCO$_2$): A measure of the levels of carbon dioxide (CO_2) in exhaled breath, which is at its maximum level at the end of expiration.

Fetal distress: A compromised condition of the fetus characterized by certain signs such as a markedly abnormal heart rate and potential passage of meconium prior to or during labour.

Laser treatment: A treatment for severe retinopathy of prematurity where lasers are applied to the outside of the retina to halt the spread of abnormal blood vessels.

Otoacoustic Emissions (OAE) test: One of two hearing screening tests undertaken by a probe placed in the ear canal that generates wide-band clicks. Measures the integrity of the inner ear.

Oxygen saturation (SpO$_2$): A measure of how much oxygen the blood (haemoglobin) is carrying as a percentage. Measured by a pulse oximeter. (See *Oxygen therapy* glossary).

Post-term: Beyond the estimated date of delivery.

Pregnancy complications: These can include: pre-eclampsia, maternal seizure, thyroid disorder, diabetes, placenta praevia, known illicit drug use, shoulder dystocia, prolapsed cord.

Preterm neonate: Baby born prematurely, before 37 completed weeks of pregnancy.

Retinopathy of prematurity (ROP): An abnormal growth of blood vessels in the eye, occurring only in preterm babies exposed to high oxygen concentrations. It can lead to the formation of scarring that can damage the retina.

Screening: The process of identifying who may be at risk of a particular disease.

Tachycardia: Rapid heart rate.

Tachypnoea: A rapid respiratory rate.

Term: 40 weeks gestation.

The Glossaries for *Breathing, Cardiovascular system care, Oxygen therapy* and *Respiratory distress* are also relevant to this topic and provide further assessment terminology.

Assessment: References

Apgar V. (1953). A proposal for a new method of evaluation of the newborn infant. *Current Researches in Anesthesia and Analgesia.* 32: 260–267.

Ballard, J.L. (n/d). Ballard tool for assessing gestational age http://www.ballardscore.com/

Castrodale, V. and Rinehart, S. (2014). The golden hour: Improving the stabilization of the very low birth-weight infant. *Advances in Neonatal Care.* 14 (1): 9–14.

Chalmers S. and Mears M. (2005). Neonatal pre-transport stabilisation – Caring for infants the STABLE way. *Infant.* 1 (1): 34–37.

Bissinger, R. and Annibale, D. (2010). Thermoregulation in very-low-birth-weight infants during the golden hour: Results and implications. *Advances in Neonatal Care.* 10 (5): 230–238.

Doyle, K.J. and Bradshaw, W.T. (2012). Sixty golden minutes. *Neonatal Network.* 31 (5): 289–294. doi: 10.1891/0730-0832.31.5.289.

Hazinski, M. (2012). *Nursing Care of the Critically Ill Child (3rd edition).* London and New York; Elsevier.

International Committee for the Classification of Retinopathy of Prematurity (2005). The International Classification of Retinopathy of Prematurity revisited. *Arch Ophthalmol.* 123 (7): 991–999.

Lomax, A. (ed.) (2011). *Examination of the Newborn; An Evidence Based Guide.* Chichester: Wiley Blackwell.

NHS National Screening Committee. (2015) http://newbornphysical.screening.nhs.uk

NHS Newborn Bloodspot Screening (2015) http://newbornbloodspot.screening.nhs.uk/

NHS Newborn Hearing Screening Programme http://www.nhsp.info/

National Institute for Clinical Excellence. (NICE, 2013). CG 160 Feverish illness in children; NICE Guidance http://guidance.nice.org.uk/CG160/NICEGuidance/pdf/English

Petty, J. (2011). Fact sheet; Neonatal biology – An overview part 3. *Journal of Neonatal Nursing.* 17 (4): 128–131.

Rennie, J. and Kendall, G. (2013). *A Manual of Neonatal Intensive Care (2nd edition).* London: CRC Press.

Royal College of Nursing (RCN) (2013). Standards for assessing, measuring and monitoring vital signs in infants, children and young people. *RCN guidance for nurses working with children and young.* https://www.rcn.org.uk/__data/assets/pdf_file/0004/114484/003196.pdf

Royal College of Paediatrics and Child Health, Royal College of Ophthalmologists, British Association of Perinatal Medicine and BLISS (2008). *Guideline for the screening and treatment of retinopathy of prematurity.* http://www.bapm.org/publications/documents/guidelines/ROP_Guideline%20_Jul08_%20final.pdf

Stenson, B., Brocklehurst, P., and Tarnow-Mordi, W. (2011). Increased 36-week survival with high oxygen saturation target in extremely preterm infants. *N Engl J Med.* 364: 1680–1682.

Saugstad, O.D. and Aune, D. (2014). Optimal oxygenation of extremely low birth weight infants: A meta-analysis and systematic review of the oxygen saturation target studies. *Neonatology.* 105: 55–63.

Breathing and blood/blood taking

This chapter also covers two topics; the first is breathing comprising respiratory and ventilation management and the second is understanding blood taking and useful values.

Breathing and ventilation

A healthy baby with an open airway will be able to breathe spontaneously without problems. However, in neonatal care, respiratory management to support a neonate's breathing is often necessary. While intubation for full ventilation support may be required in the intensive care setting, this should only be done if absolutely necessary (Habre, 2010). Non-invasive means of airway and breathing support is always preferable to avoid the potential long-term damage to lungs from mechanical ventilation (Davis et al., 2009; Bellettato et al., 2011; Brown and DiBlasi, 2011). The ultimate aim is to wean any support as soon as possible and for the neonate to breathe on their own.

This section covers all ventilation strategies starting with the application of continuous positive airway pressure (CPAP) and then moving through the more invasive means of positive pressure ventilation and less conventional methods of support (Tables 2.9 – 2.14 and Boxes 2.9 – 2.11 inclusive).

> Related topics: in line with the A-B-C approach highlighted in the *Airway* and *Assessment* sections, the topic of *Breathing* follows on logically from this. Oxygen therapy, administration and monitoring are covered in the *Oxygen therapy* section.

Continuous positive airway pressure

A non-invasive respiratory support therapy is CPAP, which is administered non-invasively by a flow driver, as shown in Figure 2.4 via two short nasal prongs or a mask over both nostrils. Table 2.9 and Box 2.9 summarize CPAP, the way in which it is administered and the variety of modes available. The flow driver offers a selection of modes to avoid the need for intubation/re-intubation and to assist in weaning the neonate from mechanical ventilation. One or two (biphasic) CPAP levels can be given.

Table 2.9   Continuous biphasic positive airway pressure (BiPAP) guide –
SUMMARY TABLE

Knowledge point	Practice implication
Infant flow SIPAP® provides bi-level nasal CPAP (see Figure 2.4)	A baseline pressure is set as well as extra 'pulses' or 'sighs' (brief periods of increased pressure)
Baseline pressure, a set flow of 8–10 litres/minute (on the 'low pressure' flow dial) is set to obtain pressure	8–10 litres/minute should give a pressure of 4–6 cm/water provided that there is an adequate seal at the nostrils. Altering the flow will affect the pressure given
For additional pressure, set this using the second 'high pressure' flow dial – set at 2 litres/minute	The 'pulses' or 'sighs' of increased pressure above the baseline CPAP pressure (see Figure 2.4) may be timed, or 'triggered' by the neonate's own inspiratory efforts
A special 'flip' mechanism in the connection to the nose supports the neonate's breathing throughout both inspiration and expiration	The continuous gas flow provides a residual and stable gas CPAP pressure delivery throughout the respiratory cycle. When expiration stops, the flow instantly flips back to the inspiratory position
Modes	
CPAP	One level of pressure. It can be given with or without an 'apnoea' transducer placed onto the abdomen
Biphasic timed	A baseline pressure is set and the extra pressure supported 'sighs' are delivered according to a set 'rate' and inspiratory time
Biphasic trigger	As above but the extra pressure sighs are not timed: they are triggered by the neonate initiating a breath
Biphasic + apnoea	As for *biphasic timed* but there is additional apnoea monitoring and an alarm will sound if the neonate does not breathe within the apnoea interval (as for CPAP and apnoea above)

CPAP should always be considered before more invasive modes of intubation and full ventilation in line with a protective lung strategy (Bellettato et al., 2011; Brown and DiBlasi, 2011). ▐▶ See also *Respiratory distress* and its related management.

> **Box 2.9   Nursing care of the neonate on CPAP: specific practice points –**
> **CHECKLIST**

A balance is necessary between an adequate seal at the nose to maintain pressure and prevention of nasal trauma. This can be done by:

- Ensuring the nasal prongs/mask/bonnet are sized correctly according to guidelines
- Ensuring the bonnet to nose strapping provides secure fixation but is not too tight
- Positioning the neonate and the tubing appropriately so that it is well supported
- Regularly checking for nasal trauma. An assessment tool can be utilised such as the example below.

Signs	Score	Action
Nares appear healthy	0	No action required
Slight redness noted around nares Area appears painful to touch Some indentation noted	1	Ensure the baby is wearing the correct size hat/mask/prong as per unit guidelines and that all are correctly positioned Assess/discuss with senior nurse/registrar/consultant if a change in mask/prongs is needed or consider a change of device Document on intensive care unit (ICU) chart and in notes
Any of the following evident: • Marked indentation • Painful to touch • Tissue breakdown	2	Call senior nurse/registrar/consultant Remove mask/prongs immediately ensuring baby's breathing remains supported Decide on appropriate alternative respiratory support Document on relevant chart, in notes

(continued)

	Doctor to refer to plastic surgeons and obtain medical imaging

Source: Reprinted from Lamburne, S., An Assessment tool for infants requiring nasal continuous positive airway pressure. Infant journal, (2014). 10 (4), Pages 123–26, with permission from Infant journal and author.

Other Practice points

- Assess the neonate for any discomfort and provide measures to settle and console
- Continuous monitoring of vital signs including oxygen monitoring
- Humidification of CPAP gases is essential – ▶ see Figures 2.6 and 2.7
- Assess the need the oral/nasal suction – ▶ see Figure 2.8a
- Give regular mouth care due to potential dryness from gases
- Continue feeding while on CPAP if applicable – observe for abdominal distention – nasogastric tube should be in situ and left on free drainage if neonate is not fed OR to be aspirated before each feed and any excess gas removed

⬤ Check local guidance on setting up CPAP/BiPAP, weaning pressures and specific care of a neonate on CPAP.

References: De Paoli et al. (2008); McCoskey (2008); Broster and Ahluwalia (2009); Petty (2013a)

🖐 **Time off and weaning from CPAP pressure is decided according to individual clinical condition and ability to tolerate.**

Positive pressure ventilation

Sometimes referred to as intermittent positive pressure ventilation (IPPV), mechanical, mandatory or artificial ventilation, this term applies to the whole spectrum of ventilation modes that deliver positive pressure via an endotracheal tube (ETT) according to parameters set on a ventilator (Figure 2.5) (Broster and Ahluwalia, 2009; Petty, 2013b). Tables 2.10 and 2.11 and Box 2.10 provide an overview of ventilation modes.

Figure 2.4   CPAP flow driver (Carefusion)

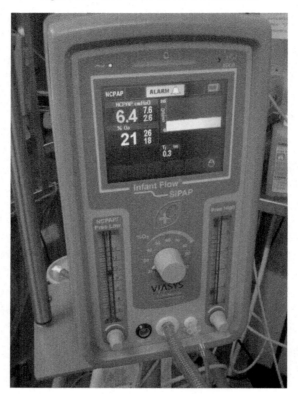

Figure 2.5   Mechanical ventilator (SLE 5000®)

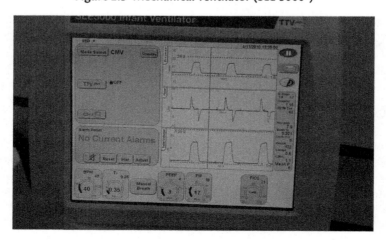

Table 2.10   A guide to ventilator modes – SUMMARY TABLE

Mode	Definition
Continuous mandatory ventilation (CMV)	Mandatory ventilation which does not allow the neonate to breathe between ventilator breaths to give maximum support. Spontaneous breathing should be minimal to avoid 'asynchrony'
Synchronized intermittent mandatory ventilation (SIMV)	SIMV synchronizes the set breaths with the neonate's breathing. A rate is set but the breaths are delivered 'in-tune' with the neonate's efforts by detecting these and synchronizing the delivery
Patient trigger ventilation (PTV)	Also called synchronized intermittent positive pressure ventilation (SIPPV) or assist control (A/C). In PTV, the neonate triggers the ventilator to deliver a breath at a set pressure and inspiratory time. Therefore the rate is determined by the neonate. A back-up rate is set
Target tidal volume (TTV) or Volume guarantee (VG)	A desired tidal volume (Vt) is set that is guaranteed and delivered at the lowest possible pressure. TTV is turned on in conjunction with an existing mode
Pressure support ventilation (PS)	In PS, breathing efforts are supported with a ventilator breath set to a desired pressure; similar to PTV but the neonate determines their own rate *and* inspiratory time (Ti). A mode in its own right or used in conjunction with SIMV where any breath that the neonate spontaneously delivers is pressure supported to a percentage of the peak pressure set
High frequency oscillation ventilation (HFOV)	A non-conventional mode of ventilation that uses breath rates or rather 'oscillations' known as frequencies, at rates much greater than normal physiological breath rates. This causes the chest to 'bounce' or vibrate
High frequency jet ventilation (HFJV)	HFJV introduces small pulses of gas under pressure into the airway at a very fast rate or frequency for a brief duration, using very small tidal volumes
Proportional assist ventilation (PAV)	PAV gives assistance that is proportional to the neonate's effort, whereby the applied pressure increases in proportion to the Vt and flow generated by the neonate, with the frequency, timing and rate of lung inflation being controlled by the neonate
Neurally adjusted ventilatory assist (NAVA)	Gas delivery from the ventilator is triggered, controlled and cycled by a diaphragmatic electromyogram (EMG) signal. The ventilator is aware of the change in EMG by the insertion of a specially designed nasogastric tube (NGT) with EMG electrodes that cross the diaphragm

(continued)

Table 2.10   Continued

NB: The actual terminology used may differ between makes and models of different ventilators

 Check local guidance on preferred ventilation modes

Source: Reprinted with permission from: Petty J. Understanding neonatal ventilation: strategies for decision making in the NICU. Neonat Netw. 2013 Jul/Aug;32(4):246–61. http://dx.doi.org/10.1891/0730-0832.32.4.246. Copyright © 2013 Springer Publishing Company, LLC.

Selecting the right mode of ventilation is determined by the neonate's condition, state of the lungs and response to existing interventions (Greenough and Donn, 2007, Hummler and Schulze, 2009; Mahmoud and Schmalisch, 2011). What is right for one neonate may not necessarily suit another.

Table 2.11   Ventilation parameters, useful formulas and definitions – SUMMARY TABLE

Parameter	Definition
Fraction of inspired oxygen (FiO$_2$)	How much oxygen is delivered – expressed as a fraction of 1. Can also be expressed as a percentage; for example, 0.3 = 30%. Oxygen is set using a dial that blends with air depending on what percentage is required
Mean airway pressure (MAP)	The total pressure (in cm H$_2$O) within the lungs throughout the respiratory cycle as determined by peak inspiratory pressure (PIP), positive end expiratory pressure (PEEP), Ti and Te. Along with FiO$_2$, this influences oxygenation (Chang, 2011) $$MAP = \frac{Rate \times I_T}{60} \times (PIP - PEEP) + PEEP$$
Tidal volume (Vt)	The volume of gas entering the lungs in one breath. Expressed in millilitres (ml). Recommended tidal volume (Vt) =4–6ml/kg
Minute volume (V$_{min}$)	The volume of gas entering the lungs over one minute expressed as litres/minute. Minute volume is tidal volume multiplied by the rate and affects CO$_2$ elimination. V$_{min}$ = Vt × rate (Chaban, 2009)
Ventilator parameters (conventional)	
Rate	The number of breaths delivered in a minute – as breaths per minute (bpm). Set by a dial or touch screen or set independently by adjusting Ti and Te (➧ see Box 2.10)

(continued)

Table 2.11   Continued

Parameter	Definition	
Peak inspiratory pressure (PIP)	The peak pressure reached at the end of inspiration (cm H_2O)	
Positive end expiratory pressure (PEEP)	The end pressure reached at the end of expiration (cm H_2O)	
Inspiratory time (Ti)	The inspiratory time of one respiratory cycle expressed in seconds. Range is 0.35–0.4 seconds	
Expiratory time (Te)	The expiratory time of one respiratory cycle expressed in seconds. With a constant or pre-determined Ti, the Te will vary depending on the required rate	
I:E ratio	The ratio of inspiration to expiration time. Te should be longer than Ti	
Flow	The flow of gas delivered. Expressed as litres per minute (l/min)	
Trigger threshold	The sensitivity of the ventilator and flow sensor to detect the neonate's breaths and trigger the ventilator	
Leak	Flow that is lost from the respiratory circuit. Measured as the difference between inspiratory and expiratory flow	
Parameters in high frequency oscillation ventilation (HFOV)		
MAP	As before – controls oxygenation along with FiO_2	
Frequency	Measured in Hertz (Hz) – 60 oscillations in 1 Hz. Set 8–10 Hz	
Amplitude	The variation around the MAP. Also known as 'delta P' or power and affects chest 'wiggle'. Controls CO_2 elimination. Set according to extent of chest wiggle/bounce and blood gas analysis	
Other ventilation terms		
Functional residual capacity (FRC)	The volume of gas present in the lung alveoli at the end of expiration	FRC is reduced in conditions such as respiratory distress syndrome (RDS) where there is poor lung compliance
Compliance	The elasticity of the respiratory system	Compliance = volume/pressure. The volume/pressure loop displayed represents the relationship graphically

(continued)

Table 2.11   Continued

Parameter	Definition	
Resistance	The capability of the airways and endotracheal tube to oppose airflow. Expressed as the change in pressure per unit change in flow	Resistance = pressure/flow Again, this is displayed graphically on some ventilators

📍 Check local guidance and model of ventilator for terminology used

Source: Reprinted with permission from: Petty J. Understanding neonatal ventilation: strategies for decision making in the NICU. Neonat Netw. 2013 Jul/Aug;32(4):246–61. http://dx.doi.org/10.1891/0730-0832.32.4.246. Copyright © 2013 Springer Publishing Company, LLC.

🖐 **It is important to learn about ventilation *terminology* in order to grasp and eventually fully understand what is observed and recorded each hour throughout the neonate's stay in intensive care.**

Box 2.10   Setting a rate using inspiratory and expiratory times – FLOW CHART

Confirm desired rate

Divide this into 60

From this figure, subtract the inspiratory time (Ti)
▽
This gives you the expiratory time (Te) that you need to set to get your desired rate

Example 1 You want a rate of 60 and Ti of 0.4 seconds
60 divided by 60 = 1 second
1 minus 0.4 = 0.6 (set the Te at 0.6 seconds)
This will give you a rate of 60
Example 2 You want a rate of 40 and Ti of 0.5 seconds
60 divided by 40 = 1.5 seconds
1.5 minus 0.5 = 1 second (set the Te at 1 second)
This will give you a rate of 40

📍 Check model of ventilator to see if the above method is used to change rate or whether a dial is used to set breaths per minute

Source: Reprinted with permission from: Petty J. Understanding neonatal ventilation: strategies for decision making in the NICU. Neonat Netw. 2013 Jul/Aug;32(4):246–61. http://dx.doi.org/10.1891/0730-0832.32.4.246. Copyright © 2013 Springer Publishing Company, LLC.

> ✋ To increase the rate while keeping the Ti the same, reduce Te.
> Conversely, to decrease the rate leaving the Ti the same, increase the Te.

Making changes to ventilation

Ventilation should be delivered in a dynamic fashion and should continually be reviewed with the aim of reducing requirements as soon as possible. Changing ventilation therefore is important to understand. Table 2.12 and Box 2.11 provide guides to changing and weaning ventilation.

Table 2.12   Changing ventilation: a guide – SUMMARY TABLE

Desired outcome	Possible actions
Conventional modes	
To increase oxygenation (increase MAP)	Increase FiO_2 (5–10%), MAP by increasing PIP or PEEP (small steps 1–2), Ti no higher than 0.4 seconds for preterm. Consider adding PSV for extra support. Consider HFOV
To decrease oxygenation when condition improves and/or during weaning (decrease MAP)	Reduce FiO_2, MAP by reducing PIP or PEEP, Ti aiming for range 0.36–0.4 seconds for the preterm neonate. Stop PSV if this has been added. Change mode to a synchronized (trigger) mode
To clear more CO_2 CO_2 elimination will be improved by increasing V_{min} (i.e. increasing the rate, Vt or both)	Increase rate (5–10 bpm) to increase V_{min}, PIP (in steps of 1–2 cm H_2O) Reduce PEEP; Note – this may cause a reduction in oxygenation, which needs to be observed. If VG (TTV) is 'on', increase desired Vt
To clear less CO_2 when weaning – CO_2 elimination will be lessened by reducing V_{min} (i.e. decreasing the rate, Vt or both)	Reduce rate in increments of 5–10 bpm, PIP (in steps of 1–2 cm H_2O) Reduce set/desired Vt if VG (TTV) is on
Oscillation	
To increase oxygenation	Increase FiO_2 in increments of 5–10% and/or MAP in increments of 1–2 cm H_2O
To decrease oxygenation when weaning	Reduce FiO_2 to an acceptable level and/or MAP in increments of 1–2 cm H_2O
To clear more CO_2	Increase amplitude (Delta P) in increments of 2–5cm H_2O according to blood gas (CO_2) and chest wiggle OR decrease frequency (Hz) allowing greater efficiency of oscillations

(continued)

Table 2.12   Continued

Desired outcome	Possible actions
To clear less CO_2 when weaning	Reduce amplitude in increments of 1–2 cm H_2O according to blood gas (CO_2) and chest wiggle

General principles: manipulating oxygenation   MAP controls oxygenation. So oxygenation can be influenced by changing any of the variables that alter MAP (PIP, PEEP, Ti and Te)   **Manipulating CO_2 elimination**   Minute volume (V_{min}) controls CO_2 elimination. CO_2 levels will be influenced by any changing measure which affects V_{min} i.e. manipulating the rate, Vt or both, will alter the V_{min} (Remember, V_{min} = Vt × rate)
Suggested actions and changes should be based on assessment of the individual neonate   Check local guidance on agreed procedures for changing ventilation   *Source*: Reprinted with permission from: Petty J. Understanding neonatal ventilation: strategies for decision making in the NICU. Neonat Netw. 2013 Jul/Aug;32(4):246–61. http://dx.doi.org/10.1891/0730-0832.32.4.246. Copyright © 2013 Springer Publishing Company, LLC.

Evaluation is an essential component of clinical decision making following any change in order to know the effectiveness of any interventions.

Box 2.11   A guide to weaning ventilation – FLOW CHART

AIM: To wean as soon as possible, in line with a protective lung strategy
▽
Is the neonate making spontaneous efforts to breath?
If no, the neonate may not be ready to wean. If yes,....
▽

CONSIDER

- Have the blood gas values normalized?
- See Table 2.12 for possible changes to ventilation during weaning in line with oxygenation or CO_2 elimination or both
- Has the oxygen requirement improved, preferably below a FiO_2 of 0.6 (60%)? Wean down oxygen as tolerated
- Has the compliance of the lungs improved, good chest expansion/lung fields?
- If on TTV/VG, is the PIP needed to reach the target volumes decreasing?
- Have any opiates/sedatives that could affect respiratory drive been stopped?
- Has the neonate been started on respiratory stimulants (caffeine)?

If no to any of these questions, the neonate may not be ready to wean.
If yes
▽
Continue to wean either pressure, rate or other parameters in
stages appropriate to the mode of ventilation. Evaluate the effect of
each change
▽
Prior to extubation, are the ventilator settings low enough to be close to the
neonate's physiological parameters (Suggestions: PIP 16–18 cm water/PEEP
4–5 cm water: MAP <10 and minimal oxygen requirement)?
▽
Extubate when appropriate based on the above requirements
▽
Following extubation, continue to assess and evaluate regularly
(Gizzi et al., 2011)

 Check local guidance on agreed procedures for changing ventilation

Source: Reprinted with permission from: Petty J. Understanding neonatal ventilation: strategies for decision making in the NICU. Neonat Netw. 2013 Jul/Aug;32(4):246–61. http://dx.doi.org/10.1891/0730-0832.32.4.246. Copyright © 2013 Springer Publishing Company, LLC.

🖐 **The intention to wean along with any weaning strategy should**
be in place as soon as a neonate is started on any means of ventilation
support, being mindful of limiting pressure, volume and oxygen.

Other care practices in ventilation

There are many areas to consider when caring for a neonate on artificial ventilation by any means. Ventilation requires gases delivered to the lungs to be warmed and humidified to prevent adverse consequences for the vulnerable airway such as drying, thickening, poor clearance of secretions and increased risk of infection. To ventilate effectively, the ETT must remain patent and regular checks should be made to ensure the adequacy of ventilation and assess the need for airway suction. Care and checking of equipment is also necessary including the flow sensor. There are of course times when other adjuncts are required in the very sick neonate such as chest drain insertion and the use of inhaled nitric oxide. The final set of tools cover these areas. They are shown in Figures 2.6–2.12, Tables 2.13–2.14 and Boxes 2.12a and b. ☛ The subject of surfactant administration is covered in *Respiratory distress*

Figure 2.6 Humidifer (Fisher and Paykel®)

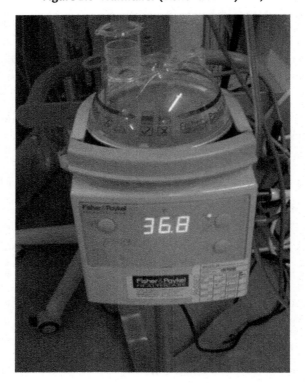

Figure 2.7 Humidification in ventilation practice – DIAGRAM

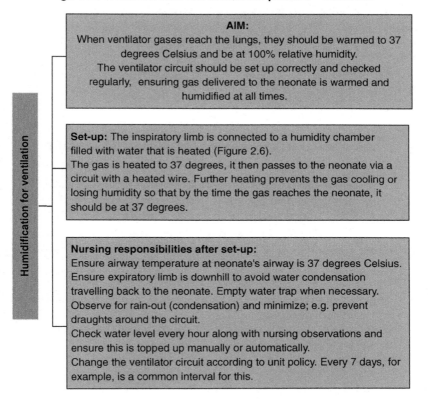

AIM:
When ventilator gases reach the lungs, they should be warmed to 37 degrees Celsius and be at 100% relative humidity.
The ventilator circuit should be set up correctly and checked regularly, ensuring gas delivered to the neonate is warmed and humidified at all times.

Set-up: The inspiratory limb is connected to a humidity chamber filled with water that is heated (Figure 2.6).
The gas is heated to 37 degrees, it then passes to the neonate via a circuit with a heated wire. Further heating prevents the gas cooling or losing humidity so that by the time the gas reaches the neonate, it should be at 37 degrees.

Nursing responsibilities after set-up:
Ensure airway temperature at neonate's airway is 37 degrees Celsius.
Ensure expiratory limb is downhill to avoid water condensation travelling back to the neonate. Empty water trap when necessary.
Observe for rain-out (condensation) and minimize; e.g. prevent draughts around the circuit.
Check water level every hour along with nursing observations and ensure this is topped up manually or automatically.
Change the ventilator circuit according to unit policy. Every 7 days, for example, is a common interval for this.

Humidification for ventilation

Check local guidance on agreed procedures for humidification set-up

Any artificial ventilation mode delivering gas to the airway and lungs must deliver warmed humidified gases to avoid any potential damage (Ho and Mok, 2003).

Suctioning the airway

Suctioning the airway is performed to maintain its patency by safe removal of secretions. In neonatal practice, suctioning can be undertaken via the nasopharyngeal (NP), oropharyngeal (OP) or endotracheal tube (ETT) route.

OP and NP suctioning: At birth it may be necessary to clear thick meconium, blood or vernix (rarely) to ensure an open airway during the early minutes of life when breathing is being established. In the case of the non-ventilated neonate in the unit, suction may be required to clear copious, thick oral or nasal secretions when they are unable to clear these themselves; for example, during a chest infection or when receiving nasal CPAP. Figure 2.8a depicts the practice points relevant for suctioning the oral and/or nasal route.

ETT suctioning: This can be performed when indicated to clear secretions and prevent a blocked tube. Figure 2.8b, Table 2.13, and Boxes 2.12a–b cover various elements of ETT suctioning in practice.

Figure 2.8a Oral and nasopharyngeal suction – FLOW CHART

Assess the *need* for suction and refer to care plan/documentation
Diminished chest movement? Increased oxygen requirement?
Increased visible and/or audible secretions?
Any previous suctioning required? Frequency?

Select appropriately sized catheter

At birth or in an emergency: use a Yankeur sucker or *no less than* an 8 to 10 fr (depending on size/gestation)
Neonatal period: use 4 to 10 fr depending on size/gestation that should be passed freely without resistance

At birth	In the neonatal period
• Suction under direct vision only using a light source to visualize the OP • Newborn resuscitation guidelines recommend a laryngoscope blade to depress the tongue down and view the back of the OP • Do not suction further than what is visualized	• Suctioning should not be done blindly • A catheter should be passed into the mouth or nose just to the back of the OP or NP but no further • No force should be applied • Withdraw catheter once inserted and apply suction *when drawing back only* taking no more than 5 seconds as a general rule

Observe and monitor throughout the procedure

 Check local guidance

Suctioning by any route is associated with potential complications (Puchalski, 2007) that include stimulation of gag reflex (OP or NP suction) sudden fluctuations in oxygenation status, hypoxia, bronchospasm, bradycardia and tissue or tracheal damage, which may not be well tolerated by fragile preterm neonates. Suctioning should be carried out with these potential risks in mind.

Figure 2.8b Endotracheal tube (ETT) suction – FLOW CHART

Assessment:
As for Figure 2.8a-
Assess the *need* for suction and refer to care plan/documentation
Consider:
Diminished or uneven chest movement? Increased oxygen requirement? Audible secretions?

Preparation:
Suction catheter of **correct size** which should not completely occlude ETT (half the size).
Open end of package and connect end of catheter to tubing.
See Table 2.13 for catheter sizing.
Measure length from end of ETT manifold to the end of the ETT
Suction checked (at 50–100 mmHg) and 'on'.

Open suction method
1. Wash hands/use sterile gloves
2. Remove suction catheter from packet and hold in sterile glove
3. Use other hand to remove manifold from ETT when the neonate is stable
4. Insert end of suction catheter into the open ETT manifold

Closed suction method
As for open suction method for steps 1 and 2.
Insert catheter end into closed suction port/adaptor on ETT manifold

Both methods:
Advance catheter down ETT for the measured distance.
Draw back and apply suction *on withdrawal only*

Assess secretions obtained
Assess neonate's response
Consider if there is a need for a repeat suction attempt (2 maximum)

Check local guidance

Suction by any route should not be done routinely and must be carried out with caution, following assessment of the neonate's clinical condition (Gardner and Shirland, 2009). Assessment should determine the frequency of the procedure tailored to the individual neonate.

Table 2.13   Suction catheter sizing – SUMMARY TABLE

ETT diameter	Catheter size
2.0 mm	4 FG
2.5 mm	5 FG
3.0 mm	6 FG
3.5 mm	7 FG
4.0 mm	8 FG

ETT suction actually occludes the airway for a given period. Therefore, it should be done swiftly and smoothly, lasting less than 5 seconds, with an appropriately sized catheter.

Box 2.12a   Suctioning with a flow sensor in place – FLOW CHART

Step 1. Set the ventilatory mode to Standby
▽
Step 2. Remove the ETT manifold from the flow sensor
▽
Step 3. Remove the flow sensor from the ETT
▽
Step 4. Carry out endotracheal suctioning
▽
Step 5. Re-fit the flow sensor to the ETT
▽
Step 6. Re-fit the ETT manifold to the flow sensor
▽
Step 7. Re-start the ventilation mode
▽

Reference: SLE® Ventilator Guidelines

Note: See Figure 2.10 for flow sensor

Suctioning of the ETT can be done via a closed system or by disconnecting the ETT from the ventilator manifold (open). The former is preferred to avoid loss of ventilator connection and support. However, with a flow sensor in place, disconnection is necessary and so the procedure should be done in the correct order as efficiently as possible.

Box 2.12b   Suctioning: additional practice points – CHECKLIST

- Due to potential complications associated with disconnecting the neonate's ventilator, *closed* suctioning is the preferred method and has been shown to have short-term benefits (Taylor et al., 2011)
- Pre-oxygenation has also been shown to assist in maintaining oxygenation (Pritchard et al., 2001) and can be considered. However, this should not be routine and oxygen can be increased by generally no more than 5–10% prior to suctioning.
- Routine normal saline (0.9%) instillation prior to suction is not supported by evidence. Consideration can be given when secretions are very thick, purulent and hard to clear
- If secretions are thick, ensure adequate humidification is being delivered by the ventilation or CPAP circuit. ☞ See Figure 2.7
- Suctioning pressures should be within the range 50–100 mmHg as a general rule

Care must be taken during suction not to introduce infection by using aseptic non-touch technique and sterile gloves. Ensure that each catheter used is inserted once only (single use) and discarded.

Check local guidance on suctioning methods and frequency for any route

References: Akgul and Akyolcu (2002); Puchalski (2007); Gardner and Shirland (2009); Pritchard et al. (2001); Taylor et al. (2011)

Individual unit variations exist on all the above points including measuring the length of the catheter insertion, closed or open suctioning methods, pre-oxygenation and instillation of saline.

Figure 2.9 Calibration of the flow sensor – FLOW CHART

Note: The flow sensor situated on the connection between the ventilation tubing and the top of the ETT (the manifold) (see Figure 2.10) is designed to measure certain parameters which are then displayed in various forms on the ventilator screen. It is important to calibrate the flow sensor prior to use and then to re-calibrate each day thereafter or when there is any circuit or ventilator change

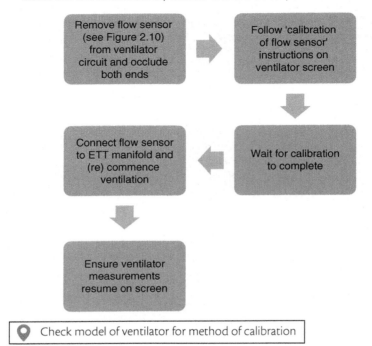

Remove flow sensor (see Figure 2.10) from ventilator circuit and occlude both ends

➡ Follow 'calibration of flow sensor' instructions on ventilator screen

⬇

Wait for calibration to complete

⬅ Connect flow sensor to ETT manifold and (re) commence ventilation

⬇

Ensure ventilator measurements resume on screen

📍 Check model of ventilator for method of calibration

Figure 2.10 Flow sensor

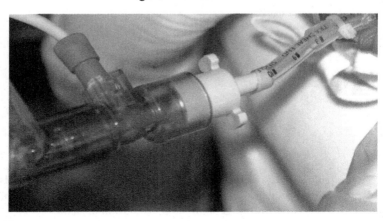

✋ It is important that flow sensors are properly and regularly calibrated to ensure accuracy of measurements.

Chest drain care

Chest drain insertion is undertaken to remove unwanted air in the presence of an air leak such as a pneumothorax or to drain fluid in the case of a pleural effusion. Diagnosis of air leak is carried out using either a cold light (chest transillumination) or definitively by chest X-ray. Figures 2.11 and 2.12 outline a chest drain set up and guidelines for assisting with the procedure.

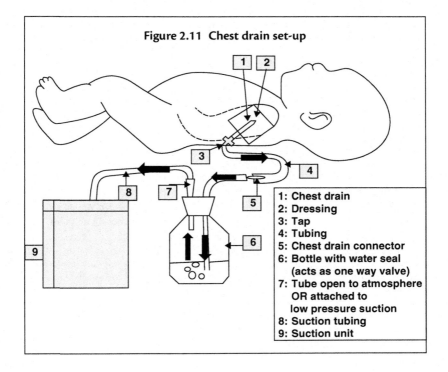

Figure 2.11 Chest drain set-up

1: Chest drain
2: Dressing
3: Tap
4: Tubing
5: Chest drain connector
6: Bottle with water seal
   (acts as one way valve)
7: Tube open to atmosphere
   OR attached to
   low pressure suction
8: Suction tubing
9: Suction unit

Figure 2.12 Assisting with chest drain insertion and care – FLOW CHART

What you need to prepare	Nursing care during chest drain insertion	Nursing Care following insertion
Chest drain kit to include water seal bottle / container Sterile water to correct level (provides the water seal 1 way valve) Chest drain tube of correct size and chest drain connector 3 way tap Blade, suture and forceps Non-occlusive dressing Low pressure suction and tubing Skin cleansing fluid and gauze Local anaesthetic and analgesia prescribed 2 chest drain clamps	Ensure analgesia and local agents have taken effect. Assist to lay out sterile field Observe vital signs / colour of the neonate at all times Once the chest drain has been inserted, a connector will be attached to the luer lock end (including a 3 way tap if necessary) Hand the tapered end of the chest drain system to the doctor / ANNP to insert into the chest drain connector This is now a closed system	Ensure the stitch / non-occlusive dressing has secured the drain Check the chest drain bottle is below the level of the neonate at all times, one end attached to the chest drain connector, the other to suction unit (low suction at 5-10 mmHg) Ensure the drain is patent at all times and the water is bubbling Never allow the chest drain bottle to be above the neonate unless clamped for a very short period only

○ Check local guidance for chest drain equipment and method of securing

The chest drain procedure is undertaken using strict aseptic technique and there are key nursing responsibilities before, during and after the procedure to maintain optimum safety and comfort of the neonate.

Tension pneumothorax is an emergency situation: ensure access to the cold light source and equipment for rapid 'butterfly' aspiration of gas prior to chest drain set-up. In addition, insertion of a chest drain is an extremely painful and invasive procedure – therefore adequate and timely pain relief must be prescribed and administered.

Inhaled nitric oxide

Finally in this section, Table 2.14 outlines the use of inhaled nitric oxide (iNO). This type of therapy can be considered medically necessary for hypoxic respiratory failure associated with evidence of persistent pulmonary hypertension of the newborn (PPHN) to improve oxygenation index (Soll, 2009). Evidence suggests that inhalation of nitric oxide at 20 parts per million (ppm) has been found to be effective in most neonates and is the standard starting dose followed by titration and weaning (DiBlasi et al., 2010). iNO is generally administered over a maximum period of 5 days (Dewhurst et al., 2007).

Table 2.14   Inhaled nitric oxide nursing guide – SUMMARY TABLE

Safety aspects	Rationale
Nurses must be trained in the set up and use of nitric oxide (NO).	The set up for giving iNO therapy involves integration of the gas into the inspiratory limb of the ventilator circuit as well as a sampling monitor attached to the circuit. Neonates are sensitive to iNO and will deteriorate quickly with sudden discontinuation – this may cause rebound pulmonary hypertension.
A backup NO cylinder should be available with an emergency manual ventilation system attached.	
Every effort should be made to avoid disconnection.	
Closed circuit suctioning should be initiated by an adaptor added to the ETT manifold.	
Monitoring	**Rationale**
Monitor oxygen requirement and the pre- and post-ductal saturation difference. Oxygenation index can also be calculated. (☞ See *Oxygen therapy*.)	Response to iNO is indicated by reduction in oxygen requirement (FiO_2 and/or oxygenation index) and pre- and post-ductal saturation difference normalizing. Toxic effects include; increased airway reactivity, altered surfactant chemistry, epithelial hyperplasia, inflammation, pulmonary oedema and production of methaemoglobin, a by-product of iNO metabolism. Methaemoglobin cannot carry oxygen.
Hourly blood gases should be taken when treatment is first commenced as part of assessing response. Four hourly blood gases should subsequently be satisfactory if the neonate is stable on treatment unless clinically indicated.	
Methaemoglobin should be checked 8–12 hourly.	
The NO and nitrogen dioxide (NO_2) levels should be continuously monitored and documented.	
Weaning iNO	**Rationale**
iNO is started at 20 ppm.	Weaning from iNO should be considered when a neonate shows clinical improvement and when oxygen requirement starts to reduce.
Neonates should be weaned to 5 ppm as quickly as possible, as long as their condition allows, preferably within 24 hours of starting therapy.	

(continued)

Table 2.14   Continued

Weaning iNO	Rationale
iNO is decreased in increments, for example between 1–2 ppm every 1–4 hours until iNO administration is 5 ppm. If weaning is difficult to this point, consider subsequent hourly decrements of 1 ppm (from 5 ppm to 1 ppm).	A neonate may not respond favourably to being weaned too rapidly from iNO; therefore, an incremental reduction is preferred.
Discontinue iNO from either 5 ppm or 1 ppm, depending on the ease of weaning.	

 Check local guidance for setting up and weaning iNO

References: Dewhurst et al. (2007); Soll (2009); DiBlasi et al. (2010)

 As for ventilation, iNO should be weaned and discontinued as soon as possible once a response is ascertained, titrated to the response of the neonate (DiBlasi et al., 2010).

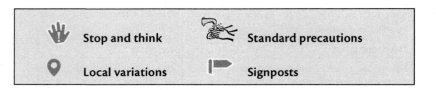

 Stop and think   Standard precautions

 Local variations   Signposts

 Always apply standard precautions when setting up and administering any mode of ventilation.

The space below can be used to record any local variations and practice points specific to your own unit.

Breathing: Glossary

Biphasic continuous positive airway pressure (CPAP or 'BiPAP'): Two alternating levels of continuous pressure are delivered to the neonates' lungs (see CPAP below).

Calibration: To check, adjust, or determine a measuring instrument by comparison with a standard. Can also be called 'zeroing.'

Chest drain: A flexible plastic tube that is inserted through the chest wall and into the pleural space used to remove air or fluid.

Continuous positive airway pressure (CPAP): A constant positive pressure, either set at one level or two alternating levels (biphasic), is applied to the airway of a spontaneously breathing neonate to maintain adequate functional residual capacity within the alveoli and prevent atelectasis.

Conventional ventilation: A range of invasive ventilation modes that aim to mimic as closely as possible the tidal breathing (inspiration and expiration) of a normal breathing pattern.

Extubation: Removal of an endotracheal tube from a neonate's airway when they are ready to come off full ventilation support following weaning.

High-frequency oscillatory ventilation (HFOV): A non-conventional form of mechanical ventilation using rates or 'frequencies' higher than normal physiological breath rates. The frequencies and power delivered make the chest 'bounce' or oscillate very quickly.

Humidification: The process of increasing the humidity of the atmosphere or, in this context, in the gas delivered in a circuit. Humidity is the presence of water vapour in a gas.

Mechanical ventilation: Using a ventilator to provide full positive pressure respiratory support of a neonate in the intensive care area until they are able to breathe for themselves.

Nitric oxide (inhaled): (iNO). A gas naturally produced by the body that can be given to help to vasodilate blood vessels within the lungs when the pressure remains high at birth following compromise and hypoxia.

Pressure controlled ventilation: Pressure controlled ventilation provides a set inspiratory pressure to deliver the gas in the inspiratory phase and passive exhalation. The amount of volume needed to deliver the breath will vary.

SiPAP® – The trade name for biphasic CPAP where two alternating levels of pressure are delivered to the neonate via nasal prongs.

Ventilator: Mechanical breathing machine used to provide artificial ventilation to a sick neonate with respiratory compromise/difficulties.

Volume controlled ventilation: Volume controlled ventilation provides a set volume of gas for the inspiratory phase with passive exhalation by the neonate. The amount of pressure needed to deliver the breath will vary.

All definitions of specific ventilation modes and terminology for relevant parameters are outlined in previous tools (Table 2.10 and 2.11). In addition, the glossaries *Airway, Assessment, Oxygen therapy* and *Respiratory distress* are also relevant to this topic and provide further terminology.

Breathing: References

Akgul, S. and Akyolcu, N. (2002). Effects of normal saline on endotracheal suctioning. *J Clin Nurs*. 11: 826–830.

Bellettato, B., Carlo, W., Rosenkrantz, T., Carter B.S., and Windle, M.L. (2011). *Assisted Ventilation of the Newborn*. http://emedicine.medscape.com/article/979268-overview

Broster, S.C. and Ahluwalia, J.S. (2009). Overview of assisted ventilation of the newborn. *Paediatrics and Child Health*. 19 (12): 537–543.

Brown, M.K. and DiBlasi, R.M. (2011). Mechanical ventilation of the premature neonate. *Respiratory Care*. 56 (9): 1298–1313.

Chaban, B. (2009). *Invasive Neonatal Ventilation*. http://pdfcast.org/download/neonatal-ventilation.pdf

Chang, D.W. (2011). *Respiratory care calculations (3rd edition)*. Albany: Delmar publ.

Davis, P.G., Morley, C.J., and Owen, L.S. (2009). Non-invasive respiratory support of preterm neonates with respiratory distress: Continuous positive airway pressure and nasal intermittent positive pressure ventilation. *Semin Fetal Neonatal Med*. 14 (1): 14–20.

De Paoli, A.G., Davis, P.G., Faber, B., and Morley, C.J. (2008). Devices and pressure sources for administration of nasal continuous positive airway pressure (NCPAP) in preterm neonates. *Cochrane Database of Systematic Reviews*. Issue 1. Art. No.: CD002977.

Dewhurst, C., Harigopal, S., and Subhedar, N. (2007). Recent advances in inhaled nitric oxide therapy in neonates: A review of the evidence. *Infant*. 3 (2): 69–75.

DiBlasi, R.M., Myers, T.R., and Hess, D.R. (2010). Evidence-based clinical practice guideline: Inhaled nitric oxide for neonates with acute hypoxic respiratory failure. *Respir Care*. 55 (12):1717–1745.

Gardner, D.L. and Shirland, L. (2009). Evidence-based guideline for suctioning the intubated neonate and infant. *Neonatal Network*. 28 (5): 281–302.

Gizzi, C., Moretti, C., and Agostino, R. (2011). Weaning from mechanical ventilation. *Journal of Maternal-Fetal and Neonatal Medicine*. 24 (S1): 61–63.

Greenough, A., and Donn, S.M. (2007). Matching ventilatory support strategies to respiratory pathophysiology. *Clinics in Perinatology*. 34 (1): 35–53.

Habre, W.A. (2010). Neonatal ventilation. *Best Practice & Research Clinical Anaesthesiology*. 24 (3): 353–364.

Ho, T. and Mok, J. (2003). Condensate clearance from CPAP circuit: An examination of two methods of draining condensate from the inspiratory tubing. *Journal of Neonatal Nursing*. 9 (4): 117–120.

Hummler, H.A. and Schulze, A.A. (2009). New and alternative modes of mechanical ventilation in neonates. *Seminars in Fetal & Neonatal Medicine*. 14 (1): 42–48.

Lamburne S. (2014). An assessment tool for infants requiring nasal continuous positive airway pressure. *Infant*. 10(4): 123–26.

Lamburne, S. (2015). An assessment tool for babies requiring nasal CPAP and high flow. *Journal of Neonatal Nursing*. 21: 2–4.

Mahmoud, R.A. and Schmalisch, G. (2011). Modern mechanical

ventilation strategies in newborns: A review. *Technology and Health Care*. 19 (5): 307–318.

McCoskey, L. (2008). Nursing care guidelines for prevention of nasal breakdown in neonates receiving nasal CPAP. *Advances in Neonatal Care*. 8 (2): 16–124.

Petty, J. (2013a). Understanding neonatal non-invasive ventilation. *Journal of Neonatal Nursing*. 19: 10–14.

Petty, J. (2013b). Understanding neonatal ventilation: Strategies for decision making in the NICU. *Neonatal Network*. 32 (4): 246–261.

Pritchard, M.A., Flenady, V., and Woodgate, P.G. (2001). Preoxygenation for tracheal suctioning in intubated,

ventilated newborn infants. Cochrane Database of Systematic Reviews 2001, Issue 1. Art. No.: CD000427. Updated 2009.

Puchalski, M.L. (2007). Should normal saline be used when suctioning the endotracheal tube of the neonate? http://www.medscape.com/viewarticle/552862

Soll, R.F. (2009). Inhaled nitric oxide in the neonate. *J Perinatol*. 29 Suppl. 2: S63–67.

Taylor, J.E., Hawley, G., Flenady, V., and Woodgate, P.G. (2011). Tracheal suctioning without disconnection in intubated ventilated neonates. Cochrane Database of Systematic Reviews. Issue 12. Art. No.: CD003065.

Blood and blood taking

Sampling blood by varying means for analysis, screening and/or diagnosis is a very common practice in neonatal care. It is therefore important to understand normal blood parameters.

Tables 2.15–2.17 and Boxes 2.13–2.16 outline normal values and ranges for the common blood tests taken in the neonatal unit including an overview of blood sampling and transfusion.

Understanding blood values specific to the neonatal group is important as there are some physiological differences in this group compared to the older child and adult.

Related topics: See also *Assessment* and place this section into the wider context of assessment as a whole. *Infection* and *Jaundice* also contain further specific information about blood analysis for these specific reasons.

As for vital signs assessment, the frequency of taking blood for the various tests that may be necessary should be decided on an individual basis.

Table 2.15   Blood values in the neonate – CHECKLIST

Parameter measured	Normal values
Albumin	33–47 g/l
Alkaline phosphatase (0–2 years)	100–350 U/l
Ammonia	<40–50 micromol/l
Amylase	8–85 U/l
Aspartate transaminase (AST)	15–45 U/l
Bicarbonate	18–25 mmol/l
Bilirubin (total)	2–24 micromol/l
Bilirubin (conjugated)	up to 4 micromol/l
C Reactive Protein (C.R.P)	<2 mg/l (although a trend is most important)
Calcium (ionized)	1.2–1.3 mmol/l
Calcium (total)	2.1–2.6 mmol/l
Chloride	9–110 mmol/l
Creatinine	60–120 micromol/l
Globulin	17–38 g/l
Glucose	3.6–5.4 mmol/L
Insulin	<15 mu/l
Iron	9–27 micromol/l
Lactate (venous)	1–1.8 mmol/l
Magnesium	0.7–1 mmol/l
Phosphate	1.3–2.1 mmol/l
Plasma osmolarity	270–295 mmol/kg
Potassium	3.5–5.5 mmol/l
Protein (total)	57–80 g/l
Sodium	135–145 mmol/l
Urea	1.0–8.5 mmol/l

Full blood count values			
Term infants			
	Cord blood	**24 hours**	**1 week**
Mean Haemoglobin (Hb) (g/dl)	16.8	18.4	17

(continued)

Table 2.15   Continued

Term infants

	Cord blood	24 hours	1 week
Range White Blood Cells (WBC) (x10/9/l)	10–26	14–31	6–15
Platelets (x10/9/l)		150–400	

Preterm infants

	Cord blood	24 hours	1 week
Mean Hb (g/dl)	14.5	15–17	17–20
Range WBC (x10/9/l)	5–19	5–21	6–18
Platelets (x10/9/l)		100–350	

	28 wks	34 wks	Term	Day 1	Day 3	Day 7	Day 14
Hb (g/dl)	14.5	15	16.8	18.4	17.8	17	16.8
PCV* %	45	47	53	58	55	54	52

*PCV (packed cell volume) mean at birth: 45–55%

General ranges for year 1 of life (after the neonatal period)

PCV	35–45%
Haemoglobin	9–14.5 g/dl
Platelets	150–400 × 10/9/l
White cells	6–18
Neutrophils	2–8.5
Lymphocytes	1–5–4
Monocytes	0.2–0.8

All the above values are averages and variations exist around the mean.
(Skinner, 2005; Rennie, 2012). Values also vary depending on age and gestation so refer to laboratory reference ranges for individual blood results.

Clotting values

Term

Test (seconds)	Day 1	Day 5	Day 30	Adult
Prothrombin time (PT)	13	12.4	11.8	12.4
Partial thromboplastin time (PTT)	42.9	42.6	40.4	33.5
Fibrinogen (g/l)	2.83	3.12	2.7	2.78

(continued)

Table 2.15   Continued

Preterm

Test (seconds)	Day 1	Day 5	Day 30	Adult
Prothrombin time (PT)	13	12.5	11.8	12.4
Partial thromboplastin time (PTT)	53.6	50.5	44.7	33.5
Fibrinogen (g/l)	2.43	2.8	2.54	2.78

(NB: Values are averages and variations around the mean exist by + or − 1–1.5 seconds) (Rennie, 2012)

Summary	
PT	12–18 seconds
PTT	29–52 seconds
Fibrinogen	1–8–4 g/l
(Skinner, 2005)	

Key: l=litre/   u= unit/   mu= microunits/   mmol= millimol/   g = gramme

🔘 Check local guidance and individual reference ranges when interpreting blood values for each neonate.

Blood gas analysis

A vital and common investigation for assessment of the sick or compromised neonate in clinical care is blood gas analysis which gives valuable information regarding a neonate's respiratory, oxygenation and metabolic status along with the response to ventilation changes, administration of oxygen and fluid (Brown and Eilemann, 2006; Armstrong and Stenson, 2007). Table 2.16 and Box 2.13 outline blood gas analysis and values.

🖐 **Remember that exceptions to 'normal', 'text-book' values apply, depending on the individual situation, for example, permissive hyper-capnia, compensated values, site of sampling. These must be considered in the interpretation of blood gases (Farmand and Nash, 2009).**

Table 2.16   Blood gas values in the neonatal unit – SUMMARY TABLE

	pH	CO₂	O₂	Bicarbonate	Base
Cord (arterial)	7.25–7.28	48 mmHg 6.5 kPa	18–22.5 mmHg 2.4–3 kPa	n/a	−4
Cord (venous)	7.28–7.35	35–45 mmHg 5–6 kPa	27–38 mmHg 3.8–5 kPa	n/a	−4
Neonatal (arterial)	7.35–7.45	35–45 mmHg 4.6–6 kPa	50–90 mmHg 7–12 kPa Term 50–80 mmHg 6.5–10.5kPa Preterm	22–26 mEq/l Term 20–24 mEq/l Preterm Or 22–26 mmol	+2 to −2

For 'Uncompensated' gas (i.e. pH is abnormal)

Low pH and high CO₂ = respiratory acidosis

Low pH and large base deficit/low bicarbonate = metabolic acidosis

High pH and low CO₂ = respiratory alkalosis

High pH and large base excess/high bicarbonate = metabolic alkalosis

Low pH, high CO₂ and large base deficit = mixed acidosis

For 'compensated' gas (i.e. pH is normal but other values are out of range)

pH	CO₂	Bicarbonate	Problem
Low normal	High	High	Compensated Respiratory acidosis
High normal	Low	Low	Compensated Respiratory alkalosis
Low normal	Low	Low	Compensated Metabolic acidosis
High normal	High	High	Compensated Metabolic alkalosis

 Check local guidance on agreed/acceptable blood gas norms and ranges

Source: Reprinted with permission from: Petty J. Understanding neonatal ventilation: strategies for decision making in the NICU. Neonat Netw. 2013 Jul/Aug;32(4):246–61. http://dx.doi.org/10.1891/0730-0832.32.4.246. Copyright © 2013 Springer Publishing Company, LLC.

Consider the following additional notes.

Permissive hypercapnia. Accept different values to the normal range outlined previously. To avoid over-ventilating the lungs, keep pH >7.25. Watch base deficit and keep between −4 to +4.

kPa or mmHg? Values are expressed in both kPa *and* mmHg for PaO_2/$PaCO_2$ *and* in mEq/l *and* mmol for bicarbonate to account for differences between countries.

Arterial, capillary or venous? Arterial blood is preferred for most accurate blood gas values. Capillary and venous neonatal sampling can be considered for all values (pH, CO_2, base and bicarbonate) *except oxygenation status*.

Box 2.13   Interpretation of blood gases in the neonatal unit – FLOW CHART

1 Assess pH
(Is the pH normal? If not, is it acidotic or alkalotic? See values)

2 Assess respiratory component
Is CO_2 within normal range?
▽
3 Assess metabolic component
Is the bicarbonate within normal range and is there a large base deficit or excess?
▽
4 Assess if compensation has occurred
i.e. has the pH normalized but the other values are out of normal range?

5 Assess oxygenation (PaO_2)
A low PaO_2 can contribute to a metabolic acidosis by anaerobic respiration by cells and lactic acidosis accumulation
Plus
Consider lactate levels

6 Interpret and make plan of action

7 Evaluate/Reassess

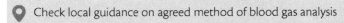
Check local guidance on agreed method of blood gas analysis

Source: Reprinted with permission from: Petty J. Understanding neonatal ventilation: strategies for decision making in the NICU. Neonat Netw. 2013 Jul/Aug;32(4):246–61. http://dx.doi.org/10.1891/0730-0832.32.4.246. Copyright © 2013 Springer Publishing Company, LLC.

A systematic approach to working through the different aspects of a blood gas analysis result is useful, always considering the pH *as a priority* and then leading on to working out what has contributed to the change in pH.

Blood glucose

Blood glucose is the main energy source essential for all bodily functions and its analysis is another common test within neonatal care. A healthy term neonate, provided they are kept warm and fed within the first few hours of birth, should be able to control their own blood glucose concentration (Petty, 2010). However, during compromise, stress or illness, a neonate may not be able to mount this normal metabolic adaptation when glucose levels drop; thereby necessitating a specific operational threshold (Hawdon, 2005); i.e. an optimum value for treatment and glucose administration. Box 2.14 addresses blood glucose monitoring.

Controversies have existed previously on what is the operational threshold for blood glucose in the treatment of hypoglycaemia; in the high risk neonate, this is now generally accepted at 2.6 mmol (Deshpande and Ward-Platt, 2005; UNICEF, 2013).

Box 2.14 Blood glucose monitoring in the neonatal unit – SUMMARY TABLE

a) Hypoglycaemia
Identify the 'at-risk' neonate

- Preterm gestation, small for gestational age, low birth weight (<2.5 kg), maternal diabetes, intrapartum compromise, resuscitation at birth, sick neonates (e.g. infection), hypothermia (Harris et al., 2012; UNICEF, 2013).

Ensure ongoing observation and documented monitoring

- Signs to observe for: altered level of consciousness, apnoea, cyanosis, hypothermia, jitteriness, convulsions, reduced tone (Cranmer et al., 2014).

Operational threshold defined as 2.6 mmol/l*

- This is the consensus based on evidence as stated above (UNICEF, 2013).
*NB: NICE (2008) state 2.0 mmol/l. However, commonly the minimum threshold for admission to the NNU is 2.6 mmols/l

 Refer to local unit policy

(continued)

The feeding neonate

- At-risk neonates who do not require intensive care should feed as soon as possible after birth (within 30 minutes) and then at frequent intervals, for example, every 2–3 hours, until feeding maintains their *pre-feed* blood glucose levels at the desired level. An example would be a neonate born to a diabetic mother
- Additional measures such as tube feeding (for 'top ups' with expressed breast milk or formula milk) or intravenous (IV) dextrose should be implemented only if necessary, such as where:
  - The blood glucose remains below threshold despite maximal support for feeding
  - Abnormal clinical signs occur
  - The neonate will not orally feed effectively

The neonate with hypoglycaemia in intensive care who is unable to feed

- IV dextrose 10% is given firstly as a bolus (2–2.5 ml/kg) followed by maintenance fluids according to the individual neonate's condition
- Higher dextrose concentrations may be required
- Regular monitoring of blood glucose (1–2 hourly until stable) and titration of IV glucose is necessary
- Any blood glucose below 1.1 mmol/l – refer as an emergency and treat immediately

Hyperglycaemia

- Preterm neonates can be prone to hyperglycaemia due to immature ability to tolerate glucose or as a biochemical sign of stress
- It is documented to keep glucose below 10–15 mmol/l (Hawdon, 2005)
- A common consensus in the evidence is that over 8 mmol/l is classed as hyperglycaemia (Rozance and Hay, 2010)
- The decision whether to treat with insulin or not, however, is determined by both blood glucose and accompanying glycosuria (>1%)

Check local guidance on acceptable glucose norms and blood glucose monitoring procedures.

Blood sampling from neonates

When sampling blood, there are numerous considerations such as the choice of access site, what blood tests are required and how much blood is needed for the necessary tests. Box 2.15 outlines a summary of important points to address when sampling blood from a neonate.

> **Box 2.15   A guide to taking blood tests: some tips and important points – CHECKLIST**

- Think: What method is appropriate? Heel prick, venepuncture or arterial line sampling?
- What blood tests are required and is the method suitable? For example, a heel prick may not be appropriate for obtaining sufficient blood for *numerous* tests. If an arterial line is in situ, this avoids frequent distress from heel pricks. Conversely, if only a blood gas is required, a heel prick may suffice rather than waiting for someone who is able and free to perform venepuncture.
- Consider the comfort of the neonate. For any method, ensure timing is appropriate for the neonate and provide comfort measures and/or procedural pain measures (sucrose, pacifier, breast milk, facilitative holding, skin to skin).
- If the heel has been repeatedly used for sampling, it may be sore which can cause further distress. Be mindful of this.
- If cannulation is performed or arterial line is inserted, take any required blood at the same time while the opportunity arises.
- Ensure the required blood quantity is obtained all at once for all necessary tests.
- However, ensure the number of times any device in the vascular system is accessed is minimised as much as possible.
- For heel prick procedure, follow the guidance from UK Newborn Screening Programme Centre (UKNSPC, 2015) in relation to heel site. See Figure 2.13
- Taking blood: Blood should be collected as quickly and smoothly as possible to prevent any clotting or haemolysis. For example, avoid prolonged squeezing of the heel which may affect the result.

Remember to wear gloves when taking and handling blood and ensure careful hand washing before and after.

Along with the national guidance for heel pricks (see above), check local guidance on blood sampling procedures

---

Caution should be exercised concerning how much blood is taken for repeat tests. This should be carefully monitored, particularly in very small neonates, whose blood volume can easily be depleted.

Figure 2.13 Heel prick correct site

- Correct position for a heel prick blood sample

- Preferred puncture
  sites:

A) For full-term and
   preterm infants

B) For infants who
   have had repeated
   heel punctures

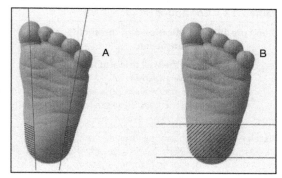

A

B

Source: Image courtesy of NHS Newborn Blood Spot Screening Programme (image adapted from Jain, A. and N. Rutter, Ultrasound study of heel to calcaneum depth in neonates. Arch Dis Child Fetal Neonatal Ed, 1999. 80(3): p. F243–5). © Crown Copyright 2013.

Note: This information was originally developed by the UK National Screening Committee/NHS Screening Programmes (www.screening.nhs.uk) and is used under the Open Government Licence v2.0.

Giving blood to neonates

A blood transfusion may be required in the neonate for the prevention of anaemia secondary to prematurity or blood loss, when the haemoglobin (Hb) drops to an operational threshold level (subject to local guidelines on low acceptable values) (Kelly and Williamson, 2013). Table 2.17 and Box 2.16 outline a guide with practice points for giving blood transfusions to neonates.

Table 2.17   A guide to giving blood products in the neonatal unit – SUMMARY TABLE

Blood product	Indication and threshold for transfusion	Monitoring
Packed cells 10–20 ml/kg	**For anaemia/blood loss** First 24 hours Hb <12 g/dl or PCV <35% **Intensive care neonate** Hb <11–12 g/dl * PCV <0.35–0.40* **High dependency neonate (CPAP)** Hb <8–11 g/dl* *Lower limits apply to those in <30% oxygen and >28 days old Higher limits apply to those in oxygen >30% and <28 days	For any blood products, baseline observations include: temperature, heart rate, respiratory rate and sometimes blood pressure. All routine neonatal monitoring should be continued Check packed cell volume (PCV)/ haemoglobin (Hb)

(continued)

Table 2.17   Continued

Blood product	Indication and threshold for transfusion	Monitoring
	In the well preterm neonate with late anaemia Transfuse if symptomatic. If reticulocytes > 1%, a transfusion may not be necessary	
Platelets 10–20 ml/kg	Thrombocytopenia Neonate who is unwell/bleeding < 30–50 (x10/9/l) Stable neonate < 20 (x10/9/l)	Check platelets
Fresh frozen plasma (FFP) 15 ml/kg	Prolonged clotting time (PTT)	Check clotting times
Cryoprecipitate 5–10 ml/kg	Low fibrinogen	Check fibrinogen

⦿ Check local guidance on agreed values and operational thresholds for blood transfusion

---

✋ **Controversies and variations in practice exist as to when neonates require blood transfusions in relation to the *operational threshold*.**

Box 2.16   Giving blood: additional practice points – CHECKLIST

Checking

There are special requirements in the prescription of blood and blood components for neonates e.g. irradiated or Cytomegalovirus (CMV) negative:

- The blood unit and compatibility slip should be checked by two nurses against the neonate's ID band. The pack should be inspected for integrity before connection to the blood transfusion giving set
- The expiry date of the blood must not be exceeded

Procedural aspects

- *Aseptic non-touch technique* (ANTT) should be utilized for connection of the transfusion
- A sterile blood transfusion giving set must be used to filter and run through the blood for administration. A sterile platelet giving set may be used for transfusion of platelets and cryoprecipitate
- Drugs must never be added to blood
- Transfusion must be completed within 4 hours

(continued)

- Blood should only be warmed using a blood transfusion warmer
- The empty bag must be disposed of according to local policy

 Remember to wear gloves and use aseptic non-touch technique (ANTT) when handling and administering blood products. Ensure careful hand washing before and after the procedure.

 Along with national guidance above, check local guidance on giving blood products.

References: British Committee Standards in Haematology (2004); UK Blood Transfusion and Tissue Transplantation Services (2013)

Any neonate receiving a blood transfusion should be monitored.

	Stop and think		**Standard precautions**
	Local variations		**Signposts**

Always apply strict standard precautions when sampling or giving any blood products

---

 The space below can be used to record any local variations and practice points specific to your own unit.

Blood and blood taking: Glossary

ABO incompatibility: Blood incompatibility between the different blood groups of mother and fetus resulting in destruction of fetal red blood cells, jaundice and anaemia.

Acidosis: An accumulation of acid in the body tissues meaning the pH is lower than the expected norm, caused by respiratory or metabolic compromise or a combination of the two.

Alkalosis: The body tissues and blood have a pH higher than the normal range. As for acidosis, it can be respiratory or metabolic in origin.

Anaemia: A deficiency of haemoglobin (Hb) in the blood.

Base: The chemical opposite of acid. Base excess and base deficit refer to a surplus or deficit respectively, in the amount of base present in the blood.

Blood gases: Levels of oxygen and carbon dioxide in the blood. A blood gas analysis in full measures pH, PaO_2, $PaCO_2$, bicarbonate and base deficit/excess (Pa = partial pressure).

Carbon dioxide: A gas formed during respiration, which is exhaled during expiration.

Clotting: A test of the coagulating ability of the blood

Coagulopathy: Any disorder requiring treatment in order to maintain or recover normal blood clotting function.

Compensation: The physiological process of adjusting for an abnormal pH by either the lungs or the kidneys.

Coombes test or direct antiglobulin test (DAT) – A test used to detect presence of antibodies or complement proteins that are bound to the surface of red blood cells indicating incompatibility has occurred.

Cross-matching: Testing the compatibility of a donor's and a recipient's blood.

Cryoprecipitate: An extract rich in a clotting factors obtained as a residue when frozen blood plasma is thawed.

Disseminated intravascular coagulopathy (DIC): Pathological activation of clotting cascade mechanisms leading to microclots in the small capillaries and bleeding. Happens in response to disease such as infection.

Fresh frozen plasma: Blood plasma that has been frozen and preserved which contains all the clotting factors and is used in coagulopathy.

Full blood count: A blood test that measures the number and status of different types of blood cells, including haemoglobin, white cells and platelets.

Glucose: Glucose provides the body with energy and is essential for all cells of the body providing the 'fuel' for respiration which generates ATP, the energy source for all cells.

Group and save: Blood test to identify ABO and Rhesus blood group and antibody profile.

Haematocrit: The packed cell volume (PCV) expressed as a percentage. Newborns have a higher haematocrit than adults and older children.

Hypercapnia: Higher than normal levels of carbon dioxide in the blood.

Hypocapnia: Lower than normal levels of carbon dioxide in the blood.

Hyperglycaemia: A whole blood glucose concentration of >8 mmol/l.

Hypoglycaemia: Blood glucose below 2.6 mmol/l.

Lactate: A by-product of anaerobic metabolism when oxygen delivery to the tissues is insufficient to support normal metabolic demands.

Operational threshold: The point or value at which treatment is considered.

Packed cells: Red blood cells collected and bagged for transfusion.

Packed cell volume: See *Haematocrit*.

Platelets: Small colourless disc-shaped cells found in blood and involved in clotting.

Polycythaemia: A condition that causes 'sluggish' circulation due to an abnormally high number of red blood cells (high packed cell volume (PCV)).

Reticulocyte: Immature red blood cell made in the bone marrow.

Rhesus (Rh) disease: Blood incompatibility as a result of a mother being Rh negative and her fetus being Rh positive. As for ABO incompatibility, this causes destruction of fetal red blood cells.

Thrombocytopenia: Low platelet count.

Urea and electrolytes: A blood test to detect abnormalities in blood chemistry including kidney function.

The Glossaries for *Infection* and *Jaundice* are also relevant to this topic and provide further explanation on specific conditions that necessitate blood sampling/tests.

Blood and blood taking: References

Armstrong, L. and Stenson, B.J. (2007). Use of umbilical cord blood gas analysis in the assessment of the newborn. *Arch Dis Child Fetal neonatal edition*. 92 (6): F430 – F434.

British Committee Standards in Haematology. (2004). Transfusion guidelines for neonates and older children. *British Journal of Haematology*. 124: 433–453.

Brown, B. and Eilemann, B. (2006). Understanding blood gas interpretation. *Newborn and Infant Nursing Reviews*. 6 (2): 57–62.

Cranmer, H. (2014). Neonatal Hypoglycemia. http:// emedicine.medscape.com/ article/802334-overview

Deshpande, S. and Ward-Platt, M. (2005). The investigation and management of neonatal hypoglycaemia. *Seminars in Fetal and Neonatal Medicine*. 10 (4): 351–362.

Farmand, M. and Nash, P. (2009). Blood gas analysis and the fundamentals of acid-base balance. *Neonatal Network*. 28 (2):125–128.

Harris, D.L., Weston, P.J., and Harding, J.E. (2012). Incidence of neonatal hypoglycemia in babies identified as at risk. *J Pediatr*. 161 (5): 787–791.

Hawdon, J.M. (2005). Blood glucose levels in infancy - clinical significance and accurate measurement. *Infant*. 2 (2): 24–27.

Kelly, A.M. and Williamson, L.M. (2013). Neonatal transfusion. *Early Human Development*. 89: 855–860.

NICE. (2008). *Diabetes in Pregnancy*. NICE: London.

Petty, J. (2010). Fact sheet: Adaptation of the newborn to extra-uterine life. Part 2; Thermoregulation and glucose homeostasis. *Journal of Neonatal Nursing*. 16 (5): 198–199.

Petty J. (2013). Understanding neonatal ventilation: strategies for decision making in the NICU. Neonat Netw. 32(4):246–61.

Rennie, J. (2012). *Rennie and Robertons Textbook of Neonatology (5th edition)*. London: Churchill Livingstone.

Rozance, P.J. and Hay, W.W. (2010). Neonatal hyperglycemia. *NeoReviews*. 11 (11): e632–e639.

Skinner, S. (2005). *Understanding Clinical Investigations – A Quick Reference Manual (2nd edition)*. London/ Philadelphia; Bailliere Tindall.

UK Blood Transfusion & Tissue Transplantation Services. (2013). *Transfusion in the neonate*. http:// www.transfusionguidelines.org.uk/ transfusion-handbook/10-effective-transfusion-in-paediatric-practice

UK Newborn Screening Programme Centre (UKNSPC). (2015). *Guidelines for Newborn Blood Spot Sampling*. http://newbornbloodspot.screening. nhs.uk/bloodspotsampling

UNICEF. (2013). *Guidance on the development of policies and guidelines for the prevention and management of Hypoglycaemia of the Newborn*. http://www.unicef.org.uk/Documents/ Baby_Friendly/Guidance/hypo_policy. pdf?epslanguage=en

Cardiovascular care and communication

This chapter covers the following two topics; cardiovascular (CVS) care and communication.

Cardiovascular system (CVS) care

A healthy neonate who has a clear airway and is breathing effectively will be well perfused with a cardiovascular system (CVS) able to deliver all essential nutrients and oxygen to the body. However, in the sick neonate who does not have the compensatory mechanisms to cope with compromise, support for the CVS is often necessary. This unit covers an overview of CVS care (Boxes 2.17a–b, 2.18a–c, 2.19a–b, and Table 2.18).

This topic area follows on logically from the A-B-C approach highlighted earlier. This is the 'C' of ABC. Refer to *Airway* and *Breathing* for the two preceding topics. There is a close relationship between all three systems. Cardiovascular care also links with *Blood and blood taking*.

Box 2.17a   Monitoring the cardiovascular system (CVS) – CHECKLIST

Practice points

CVS compromise and poor tissue perfusion is indicated by:

- Hypotension – low mean blood pressure (MBP <30 mmHg)*
- Tachycardia
- Capillary refill time >3 seconds
- Metabolic acidosis e.g. lactate >2 mmol/l and/or base deficit greater than–8 mmol/l with normal chloride.
- Oliguria <1 ml/kg/h, especially after 24 hours of age.

*A general agreement on early MBP is to consider the gestation of the neonate in weeks. Hypotension can be seen therefore as MBP being below this figure (Subhedar and Shaw, 2003). However, in practice, an MBP less than 30 mmHg is often the acceptable lower limit and giving fluid volume may be considered at this point.

References: Kent et al. (2009); Broom and Parry (2012); Dionne et al. (2012); Knight (2012); Yates and Rennie (2014).

(continued)

Monitor arterial blood pressure, heart rate, capillary refill time (CRT), blood gases (lactate and base excess) and urine output. Also, ensure adequate oxygen saturations, other blood gas values, glucose and respiratory function/lung expansion are addressed and maintained.

Monitor MBP continually via arterial line or by regular cuff readings:

🢒 See Box 2.19a and 2.19b. (Johnstone and Smith, 2008).

🖐 **Caution should be exercised when administering fluid volumes to a neonate as kidney function is immature. The risk of overload should be guarded against.**

Box 2.17b   Management of cardiovascular system (CVS) compromise – CHECKLIST

Aims: To improve/optimize cardiac output and perfusion of vital organs and to prevent shock

- Labour room resuscitation care may include respiratory support, IV volume and/or blood, sodium bicarbonate,* glucose or adrenaline
- Overall, therapeutic interventions may include volume, inotropes and/or steroids for hypotension (Dempsey and Barrington, 2007; Gupta, 2012)
- **Volume:** 10–20 ml/kg saline or blood products if there is clear evidence of blood loss e.g. Antepartum haemorrhage (APH), placental abruption, severe pallor, low PCV
- **Inotropes:** dobutamine, dopamine, (Subhedar and Shaw, 2003) or adrenaline. Avoid starting inotrope infusions at less than 0.5 ml/hr, as it will take too long for effective drug delivery to reach a stable state
- **Corticosteroids** can be considered in conjunction with the above therapies but with caution.

* Sodium bicarbonate correction (to correct a metabolic acidosis)
Full correction =
0.3 x weight in kg x base deficit = the volume of sodium bicarbonate (base) in mmol
(NB: 1 mmol = 1 ml)
Divide by 2 for half correction
Dilute 1:1 with 5% dextrose or water for injection

📍 Check local guidance on monitoring and management strategies for the CVS

🖐 The potential risks of drugs used to increase blood pressure should be considered and close monitoring undertaken. For inotrope administration, care should be taken titrating doses to avoid rapid swings in blood pressure that can affect the brain perfusion (Fanaroff and Fanaroff, 2006). Caution should be exercised with the administration of sodium bicarbonate and steroid use due to their potential serious side effects.

Cardiac failure overview

CVS care is also relevant to the neonate who presents with *cardiac failure* either from congenital heart disease (CHD) or, less commonly, from non-structural causes. Generally speaking, a neonate presenting with cardiac failure for whatever reason presents with a characteristic set of signs and symptoms requiring specific management. These areas will be covered in turn starting with an overview of congenital heart anomalies (Table 2.18) and leading to the assessment and management of cardiac failure (Boxes 2.18a –c).

Table 2.18   Classification of congenital heart anomalies –
SUMMARY TABLE

	Cyanotic
Right to left shunt	Tetralogy of Fallot Transposition of the great arteries Tricuspid atresia Pulmonary atresia Persistent truncus arteriosus Total anomalous pulmonary venous return
	Acyanotic
Left to right shunt	Ventricular septal defect Atrial septal defect Patent ductus arteriosus Atrioventricular septal defect
Obstructive conditions	Pulmonary stenosis Aortic stenosis Coarctation of the aorta Hypoplastic left heart syndrome

CHD can be life threatening and may require immediate action. In less severe cases however, it may not require intervention until later in life, or none at all.

Box 2.18a   Cardiac failure: presenting signs – CHECKLIST

Cardiac failure: initial presentation in first few days

- Heart murmurs on routine screening
- Tachycardia
- Breathlessness
- Tachypnoea
- Difficulty feeding
- Failure to thrive
- Cyanotic episodes (especially during feeding)
- Sudden collapse

Congestive cardiac failure (CCF): later presentation

- Tachycardia
- Cardiac enlargement
- Tachypnoea, intercostal retractions, grunting, flaring, dyspnoea, rales and cyanosis
- Gallop rhythm
- Mottling/decreased perfusion (prolonged capillary refill) and decreased pulses
- Decreased urine output and oedema

Differentiating cardiac from respiratory causes of heart failure is essential as soon as possible, for prompt referral and transfer to a cardiac centre if necessary (Leach, 2012).

Box 2.18b   Management overview of cardiac failure – FLOW CHART

Recognize clinical signs and symptoms (see Box 2.18a)

Diagnosis – provisional based on signs or definitive via echocardiogram/ Chest X-ray (CXR)

Request a cardiac team consultation

(continued)

Initial management

- Pre-ductal arterial blood gas (ABG) to check PaO_2 (right arm) in room air and hyperoxia test by pre- and post-ductal saturation (SaO_2) monitoring (See *Oxygen therapy*)
- Treat metabolic acidosis and poor perfusion with inotropes, fluid volume and/or sodium bicarbonate as appropriate
- Four limb BP – an upper to lower limb systolic difference of >10 mmHg is significant
- Prostaglandin E1 (PG) infusion if a duct-dependent cardiac disease is suspected

CCF

- Treat the cause (e.g. CHD or Cor pulmonale due to chronic lung disease)
- Diuretics (such as frusemide) help to decrease total body water
- Monitor vital signs.
- Watch for tachycardia, arrhythmias, decreasing SaO_2 and dyspnoea, apnoea or tachypnoea
- Maintain adequate calorific requirements

▽

Referral and transportation to tertiary centre if necessary

Check local guidance on management strategies for the cardiac neonate

Any neonate on a prostaglandin infusion should be monitored closely for potential side effects such as apnoea.

Box 2.18c   Specific application: the preterm neonate with patent ductus arteriosus – FLOW CHART

The presence of a **patent ductus arteriosus** (PDA) in a preterm neonate is due to a failure of the *ductus* to close.

Recognize clinical signs

- Signs and symptoms of congestive heart failure, increased need for oxygen and inability to wean from ventilator
- Widened pulse pressure/low diastolic pressure, bounding peripheral pulses and tachycardia with or without a gallop

▽

Diagnosis by echocardiogram

▽

- Medical management with fluid restriction and diuretics
- Continually assess pulse, heart rate, pulse pressure, perfusion, and heart auscultation for the presence of a murmur
- Indomethacin or ibuprofen administration (dosage depends on weight, gestation and renal function)
- Assess closely after indomethacin or ibuprofen for ductal closure and potential side effects
- Referral and surgery (ligation) may be necessary if medical treatment is not effective
- Teach and reassure parents.

 Check local guidance on management strategies for the neonate with a PDA

Any neonate receiving non-steroidal anti-inflammatory drugs (NSAIDs) e.g. ibuprofen, indomethacin, should be monitored closely for potential side effects such as bleeding and reduced urine output.

Blood pressure monitoring

Careful and regular assessment is necessary when the CVS is accessed by the arterial system for blood pressure monitoring of the circulation.

Box 2.19a   Monitoring arterial blood pressure in neonates – FLOW CHART

- Assist with arterial line insertion and safe securing – via umbilical artery or other peripheral arterial access. 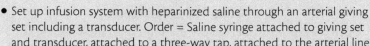 See *Umbilical care and catheters*

▽

- Set up infusion system with heparinized saline through an arterial giving set including a transducer. Order = Saline syringe attached to giving set and transducer, attached to a three-way tap, attached to the arterial line cannula

▽

- Ensure the correct waveform scale is chosen for blood pressure on the monitor

▽

- Calibrate the system to zero (see Box 2.19b below) prior to commencing monitoring

▽

- Arterial alarms should be checked on set up and at the beginning of each shift along with calibrating the transducer to zero

▽

- If there is no arterial access, take regular cuff readings hourly or as indicated by the neonate's condition, manually or automatically timed. See Table 2.6 in *Assessment* section

Standard precautions must be observed during set up of the arterial line system to prevent introduction of infection to the neonate as well as to protect oneself. The infusion fluid, transducer set and three-way tap should be changed according to local policy.

Check local guidance on blood pressure monitoring and set-up processes.

Safety: Close and regular observation of article lines should be maintained to prevent the associated risks such as bleeding, blockage by a blood clot and the effect on perfusion. Check/observe limbs for perfusion: colour, circulation, pulse and temperature of extremity distal to puncture site. The line may need to be removed if perfusion is compromised.

Box 2.19b   Procedure for zeroing an arterial line transducer – FLOW CHART

- Once the arterial line system is set up (see Box 2.19a), the transducer must constantly be level with the mid-axillary point for accuracy
- Identify the three-way tap closest to the transducer to be zeroed

Turn the tap 'off' to the neonate

Open the tap 'on' to air (remove the end-cap to allow zeroing at atmospheric pressure)

Zero the monitor according to instructions on screen

When zeroed, do the above in reverse......

Turn the three-way tap back 'off' to air by replacing the cap

Turn the tap back 'on' to the neonate

Overall, the order is ...

OFF to neonate

▽

ON to air

▽

ZERO

▽

OFF to air

▽

ON to neonate

- Observe the waveform has returned on the monitor screen and record on the observation chart

 The arterial line should be calibrated (zeroed) at the beginning of each shift or following change of neonate's position or alteration in the level of the infusion system.

 Always apply standard precautions when setting up and handling any form of arterial access. On insertion, aseptic technique is applied. Always wash hands before and after handling arterial lines and wear gloves/use aseptic non-touch technique (ANTT).

 Stop and think   Standard precautions

 Local variations   Signposts

The space below can be used to record any local variations and practice points specific to your own unit.

Cardiovascular system (CVS) care: Glossary

Capillary refill time (CRT): The time taken, in seconds, for the capillaries under the skin to refill after blanching. The time should be no more than 3 seconds in neonates.

Cardiac failure: A condition where the heart is unable to pump sufficiently to maintain blood flow to meet the needs of the body.

Cardiac output: The amount of blood pumped out by the ventricles.

Coarctation of the aorta: A congenital cardiac condition where part of the aorta is narrowed preventing adequate blood flow to the body.

Congenital heart disease (CHD): A problem with the heart's structure and function that is present at birth. Conditions can be cyanotic or acyanotic.

Cor pulmonale: Heart failure secondary to chronic respiratory compromise.

Hypertension: Higher than normal range of blood pressure.

Hypotension: Lower than normal range of blood pressure.

Hypovolaemia: A decreased volume of circulating blood in the body.

Inotrope: An agent that increases arterial tone and hence arterial pressure primarily used to maintain tissue perfusion in situations of arterial hypotension or shock.

Lactate: See Glossary *Blood and blood taking.*

Oliguria: A low urine output (<1 ml/kg/hr).

Patent ductus arteriosus (PDA): The fetal duct connecting the pulmonary artery to the aorta remains open after birth (as in preterm neonates) or can be part of a congenital cardiac defect.

Septal defects: A septal defect refers to a hole in the wall (septum) that divides the left and right sides of the heart.

Shock: An acute state in which circulatory function is inadequate to supply sufficient amounts of oxygen and other nutrients to tissues to meet metabolic demands.

Tetralogy of Fallot: A congenital cardiac condition with a combination of four heart defects, namely, pulmonary stenosis, overriding aorta, ventricular septal defect (VSD) and right sided hypertrophy (thickened muscle) of the ventricle.

Transducer: A device that converts input energy of one form into output energy of another.

Volume: The amount of blood in the circulatory system.

Transposition of the great arteries: A congenital cardiac condition where the positions of the two major arteries leaving the heart are reversed.

Zeroing: This is *calibration* of the arterial system that cancels the effects of atmospheric pressure and ensures accuracy by bringing the baseline back to zero.

The Glossaries for *Assessment* and *Blood/blood taking* are also relevant for this topic for terminology relating to blood and monitoring.

NB: Only a selection of cardiac defects have been included in this Glossary as it is beyond the remit of this book to cover the specifics of every complex anomaly.

Cardiovascular system (CVS) care: References

Broom, M. and Parry, A. (2012). The management of hypotension in the neonatal intensive care unit. *Journal of Neonatal Nursing.* 18 (6): 221–225.

Dempsey, E.M. and Barrington, K.J. (2007). Treating hypotension in the preterm infant: When and with what. A critical and systematic review. *J Perinatol.* 27: 469–478.

Dionne, J.M., Abitbol, C.L., and Flynn, J.T. (2012). Hypertension in infancy: Diagnosis, management and outcome. *Pediatr Nephrol.* 27: 17–32.

Fanaroff, A.A. and Fanaroff, J.M. (2006). Short- and long-term consequences of hypotension in ELBW infants. *Semin Perinatol.* 30: 151–155.

Gupta, S. (2012) Shock and hypotension in the neonate. http://emedicine.medscape.com/article/979128-overview

Johnstone, I.C. and Smith, J.H. (2008). Cardiovascular monitoring in neonatal intensive care. *Infant.* 4 (2): 61–65.

Kent, A.L., Meskell, S., and Falk, M.C. (2009). Normative blood pressure data in non-ventilated premature neonates from 28–36 weeks gestation. *Pediatr Nephrol.* 24: 141–146.

Knight, D. (2012) Newborn Services Clinical Guidelines: Hypotension. http://www.adhb.govt.nz/newborn/Guidelines/Cardiac/Hypotension.htm

Leach, T. (2012). Summary of congenital cardiac abnormalities. http://almostadoctor.co.uk/content/systems/paediatrics/paediatric-cardiology/summary-congenital-cardiac-abnormalities

Subhedar, N.V. and Shaw, N.J. (2003). Dopamine versus dobutamine for hypotensive preterm infants. *Cochrane Database of Systematic Reviews.* Issue 3. Art. No.: CD001242.

Yates, R. and Rennie, J.M. (2014) *Appendix 4: Normal values for neonatal blood pressure – Expert Consult.* http://www.expertconsultbook.com/expertconsult/ob/book.do?method=display&type=bookPage&decorator=none&eid=4-u1.0-B978-0-7020-3479-4..00053-2--bb0010&isbn=978-0-7020-3479-4

Communication

The principles of effective communication apply to any service user in healthcare including that between health professionals and the neonate and family (Jobe, 2010; Jone et al., 2010). Accurate verbal and written communication is an integral part of safe, good quality care (RCN, 2013). This unit covers two pertinent topics that play a central part of the daily care of the neonate: verbal handover and documentation (Figure 2.14 and Box 2.20). Handover is vital for effective verbal communication across shifts and between members of the multi-disciplinary team (MDT) (RCN, 2014). Individuals and organizations have a shared responsibility to ensure that safe continuity of information and responsibility between shift changes takes place (BMA, 2004). Documentation is legally required for all patients within the healthcare system and we have a professional duty to document clearly and maintain patient confidentiality (NMC, 2015). It is an essential part of care-planning and should comprise family needs, issues and care including, for example, any communication barriers and cultural considerations.

Figure 2.14 SBAR(D) tool for communication and handover – DIAGRAM

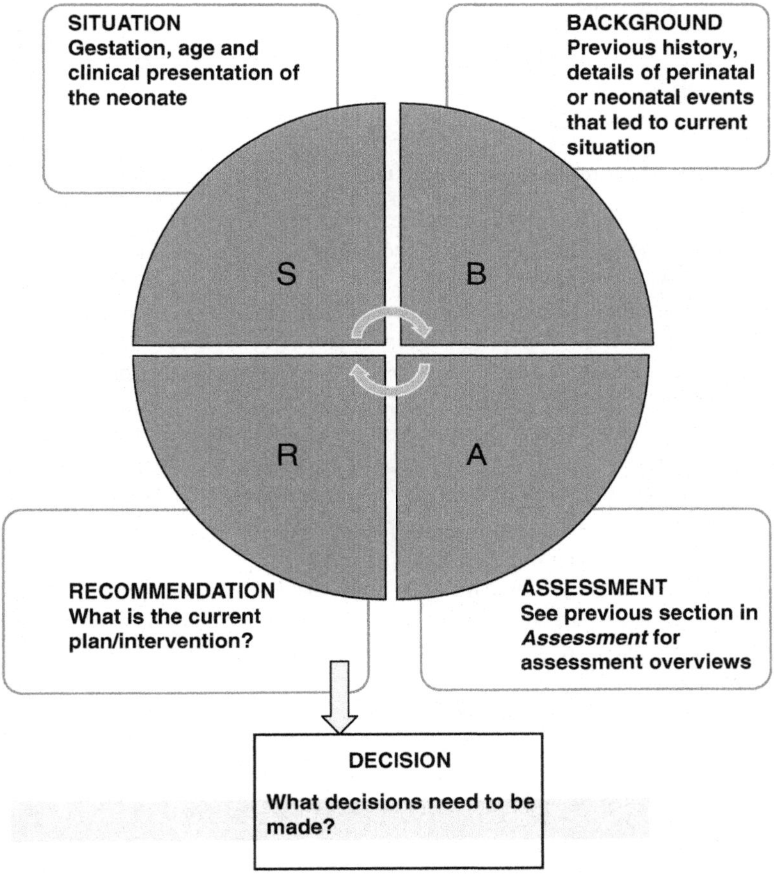

SITUATION
Gestation, age and
clinical presentation of
the neonate

BACKGROUND
Previous history,
details of perinatal
or neonatal events
that led to current
situation

S   B

R   A

RECOMMENDATION
What is the current
plan/intervention?

ASSESSMENT
See previous section in
Assessment for
assessment overviews

DECISION

What decisions need to be
made?

 Check local guidance

Source: Reference and full open access guidance from: NHS Institute for Innovation
and Improvement (2008).
(NB. SBAR was originally used in the military and aviation fields and developed for
healthcare by Dr M Leonard and colleagues from Kaiser Permanente in the USA).

Related topics: See also *Assessment* to link with the importance of docu-
menting assessment information. Documentation is also an integral component of good practice in risk management and safeguarding *(see Quality)*.
Communication is a key issue in team working *(Multi-disciplinary team)* and
for the psychological and ethical care of parents in all areas (see *Psychosocial
care of the family)*.

Handover is a key communication point to relay key information, changes and updates on both the neonate and the family.

Box 2.20   Documentation – CHECKLIST

- Communication with colleagues is essential, ensuring that they have all the information they need about the neonates and families including an individualized care plan
- Documentation should be contemporaneous, legible, and objective to be effective as a form of communication (Glasper, 2011; RCN, 2013). It should be signed with name and job title printed with a date and time on all records
- Information should be objective, accurate and the meaning clear
- It should be factual and not include unnecessary abbreviations or jargon
- All details of any assessments and reviews undertaken should be recorded. This should also include details of information given about care and treatment
- Records should identify any risks or problems that have arisen and show the action taken to deal with them
- Where appropriate, the family should be involved in the record keeping process
- The language used should be easily understood by the family
- Confidentiality- There is a need to be fully aware of the legal requirements and guidance regarding confidentiality, and practice must be in line with national and local policies. ☞ See *Psychosocial care of the family* including *Ethical-legal issues*
- Health professionals have a duty to keep up to date with, and adhere to, relevant legislation and national and local policies relating to information and record keeping
- The way information is recorded and communicated is crucial. The multi-disciplinary team (MDT) may rely on records and care plans at key communication points, especially during handover and referral.

Another essential part of documentation and communication in the neonatal unit is the formulation of individualized care plans. Care plans should document all aspects of care for the neonate and family including evaluation in line with the nursing process or any other model of planning care.

Stop and think   **Standard precautions**

 Local variations   **Signposts**

 The space below can be used to record any local variations and practice points specific to your own unit.

Communication: Glossary

Care plan: A written statement of individual assessed needs and associated planned interventions. Care planning is defined as a process that actively involves people in deciding, agreeing and sharing responsibility for how to manage their care in the neonate's case, with parents.

Contemporaneous: Meaning concurrent or 'at the same time'.

Evaluation: To appraise or view the information or outcome of an intervention in relation to its effectiveness.

Intentional rounding: Timed, planned intervention of healthcare staff in order to address common elements of nursing care, typically by means of a regular bedside ward round that proactively seeks to identify and meet patients' fundamental care needs and psychological safety.

Nursing process: A framework for nursing care involving four to six main stages – assessment, (diagnosis, outcome identification), planning, implementation and evaluation.

Objective: Impartial and actual events. Unbiased.

> The Glossaries for *Multidisciplinary team* and *Quality, risk and safeguarding* are also relevant for this topic.

Communication: References

British Medical Association (2004). *Safe handover: Safe patients. Guidance on clinical handover for clinicians and managers*. London: BMA.

Jobe, A.H. (2010.) Communication in the NICU. *The Journal of Pediatrics*. 157 (2): A2.

Jone, L., Woodhouse, D., and Rowe, J. (2010). Effective nurse parent communication: A study of parents' perceptions in the NICU environment. *Patient Education and Counseling*. 69 (1–3): 206–212.

Glasper, A. (2011). Improving record-keeping: Important lessons for nurses. *British Journal of Nursing*. 20 (14): 886–887.

NHS Institute for Innovation and Improvement (2008).

SBAR- Situation- Background- Assessment – Recommendation. http://www.institute.nhs. uk/quality_and_service_ improvement_tools/quality_ and_service_improvement_tools/ sbar_-_situation_-_background_-_ assessment_-_recommendation. html#sthash.lLY7BvjD.dpuf

Nursing and Midwifery Council (2015). *The Revised Code of Professional Conduct*. NMC: London.

Royal College of Nursing (2013). *Delegating record-keeping and countersigning records – guidance for nursing staff*. London: RCN.

Royal College of Nursing (2014). *Patient safety and human factors: RCN programme – Handover*. London: RCN.

Drugs and developmental care

This chapter covers the following two topics under 'D'; Drugs in neonatal care and Developmental care principles.

Drug administration

Comprehending the principles of drug administration is one of the core components of the Nursing and Midwifery Council's framework of nursing competency (NMC, 2010). It is an essential part of safe nursing practice to be able to calculate and administer drugs correctly and to understand their dosage, indications and side effects. This is particularly important in neonatal care as we are dealing with a distinct group of smaller, more vulnerable patients. This chapter offers guidance on some useful formulas in relation to drug units and calculations (Boxes 2.21–2.24a–c).

> Related topics: See also *Fluid balance and electrolytes* for further information on calculating doses and volumes and *Gastrointestinal care and feeding* in relation to feeding and total parenteral nutrition (TPN) calculations.

> **Neonatal drug dosages are more likely to be prescribed and given in smaller units such as micrograms than larger units, compared to older age groups. Certain drugs are also given in nanograms. It is very important to understand how to convert larger units to smaller units for accuracy and to avoid errors in administration.**

Box 2.21   Understanding strengths and units of drugs – SUMMARY TABLE

A; Converting drug units
Converting grams to milligrams to micrograms to nanograms
(multiply by 1000 to convert larger units to smaller units)

Grams (g) to milligrams (mg) – multiply by 1000
Milligrams (mg) to micrograms (mcg) – multiply by 1000
Micrograms (mcg) to nanograms (ng) – multiply by 1000

Converting nanograms to micrograms to milligrams to grams
(divide by 1000 to convert smaller to larger units)

Nanograms (ng) to micrograms (mg) – divide by 1000
Micrograms (mg) to milligrams (mcg) – divide by 1000
Milligrams (mcg) to grams (g) – divide by 1000

B; '1 in 1000', '1 in 10,000' (e.g. as used for adrenaline);
What does this mean?

(Parts of an active drug in a given volume)
1 in 1000 means 1 g in 1000 ml (1000 mg in 1000 ml = 1 mg per ml)
1 in 10,000 means 1 g in 10,000 ml (i.e. less concentrated)
1000 mg in 10,000 ml = 1 mg in 10 ml

C; Understanding millimols (mmols)
(e.g. as used for sodium bicarbonate, electrolytes)

Molarity refers to atomic weight
1 mole is the molecular weight for a drug
A mmol is one thousandth of a mole

D; Units of activity

Units are used for drugs from natural sources such as heparin
(1000 units in 1 ml), insulin (100 units in 1 ml) or hormones

E; How many grams in a certain percentage (%)

Strength as a percentage means the number of parts per hundred
5% glucose is 5 parts glucose in 100 parts of volume (5 g in 100 ml)
10% glucose is 10 parts glucose in 100 parts (10 g in 100 ml)
(Blair, 2011)

Box 2.22   Calculating drug dosages – FLOW CHART

Prior to drawing up

CHECK- Right medication, right dose, right patient, right time, and right route

How much do I need to draw up?

Volume needed =

$$\frac{\text{What you want}}{\text{What you've got}} \times \text{volume the drug is in}$$

EXAMPLE 1....

The required dose of a drug is 60 mg
The elixir contains 50 mg in 10 ml

$$\text{Volume needed} = \frac{60 \text{ mg}}{50 \text{mg}} \times 10 \text{ ml} = 12 \text{ ml (volume you need to draw up)}$$

EXAMPLE 2....

The required dose of a drug is 750 mcgs
The drug vial contains 1 mg in 1 ml

First, convert the drug concentration to the unit you wish to draw up and give, in this case mcgs.
1 mg multiplied by 1000 gives you 1000 mcgs
So, 750 mcgs divided by 1000 mcgs multiplied by 1 ml gives you 0.75 ml volume to draw up

---

You should check that both the dose prescribed and the drug being used are the same in units (e.g. milligrams) Safe prescribing is essential (Sammons and Conroy, 2008; NMC, 2010).

Drug infusion formulas

The following section gives some useful formulas for calculating drug *infusion* dosages starting with how to check how much drug is being administered from a given infusion rate.

Box 2.23   Calculating dosages from infusion rates – FLOW CHART

This should be done at the start of every shift and after infusions have been set up or changed. This formula checks what dose is being given by the infusion rate.

Quantity of drug put into syringe (in mcg or ng)*

▽

Divided by the volume in the syringe

▽

Divided by the neonate's weight**

▽

Multiplied by the infusion rate running

▽

This gives you the dose in mcg/kg/hour
(being given by the current rate of infusion)

*Convert mg to mcg first (multiply mg x 1000 to get the drug in mcg)

Or convert to ng by multiplying mg by 1000 to get mcg and then multiply again by 1000 to get ng

**NB: if the drug (e.g. inotrope) is given in mcg/kg/*minute* ALSO divide by 60 at this point **

In other words –

The initial dose (mcg) divided by the weight (kg) divided by the volume (ml) gives you *the dose **per kg per hour** in 1 ml.* You then multiply the final figure by the current rate of infusion.

Divide this by 60 (minutes) to give you the dose ***per kg per minute***

Examples

Example 1 You arrive on a shift and take over the care of a neonate who is receiving morphine via an infusion rate of 0.5 ml/hour. How much drug are they getting?

3 kg neonate on a morphine infusion

3 mg (3000 mcg) is prescribed to go into 50 ml of solution to run at 0.5 ml/hour. Work this out as follows....

3000 mcg
divided by
50 ml
divided by
3 kg

(continued)

THIS COMES TO
20 mcg/kg/hour (in 1 ml)
multiply by 0.5
gives you
10 mcg/kg/hour = dose being given

The infusion rate then changes to 0.8 ml/hour. So......
20 x 0.8 = 16 mcg/kg/hour (dose being given with new infusion rate)

Example 2 You arrive on a shift and take over the care of a neonate who is receiving dopamine via an infusion rate of 0.8 ml/hour. How much drug are they getting?
<u>2 kg neonate on a dopamine infusion</u>
90 mg (90000 mcg) is prescribed to go into 50 ml of solution to
run at 0.8 ml/hour. Work this out as follows....
90000 mcg
divided by
50 ml
divided by
2 kg
divided by
60
(**note this is an additional step compared to Example 1)
THIS COMES TO.....
15 mcg/kg/hour (in 1 ml)
15 multiplied by 0.8 gives you 12 mcg/kg/minute = dose being given
The infusion rate then changes to 0.6 ml/hr. So
15 x 0.6 = 9 mcg/kg/hour (dose being given with new infusion rate)

Check local guidance on agreed drug calculation formulas

Some drug infusions are calculated in mcg/kg/hour while others are in mcg/kg/minute depending on the half-life of the drug being given. It is important to know this when checking the prescription and to calculate accordingly.

Changing the concentration of a drug

It may be necessary to change the concentration of a drug prior to drawing up the final volume for many reasons. For example, diluting a drug (adding more volume to a given dose) changes the concentration of a drug to make the end volume larger and this assists in accuracy when drawing up very small doses.

Conversely, changing the concentration by adding more drug to a given volume is useful in relation to drug infusions when a neonate is very volume restricted, whereby the same dose can be delivered in less volume.

> Always refer to the specific drug monograph as to how a drug should be prepared, over how long it should be administered and whether it requires further dilution. For any drug, one must understand why it is being given (indication) and the associated side effects (NMC, 2010). Always check the BNF for Children (www.bnf.org/bnf/org_450055.htm) and/or local policies/drug monographs for dosage, recommended method of administration and a full list of associated side effects or contraindications (BNF, 2014).

Box 2.24a   Diluting drugs – FLOW CHART

Diluting a drug is necessary to make it _less concentrated_

Example 1 A drug which comes in a 500 mg vial which needs to be given as a 5 mg in 1 ml concentration

Example: Vancomycin. Dose required is 15 mg
Make up vancomycin 500 mg to a concentration of 500 mg in 10 ml
(which is 50 mg in 1 ml)

▽

Take out 1 ml (which is 50 mg) and put into 9 ml of normal saline or water for injection (WFI)

▽

This makes 50 mg in 10 ml which is **5 mg in 1 ml**

▽

Calculate the required dose from this 5 mg in 1 ml solution

▽

15 mg divided by 5 multiplied by 1: Volume to draw up = 3 ml

▽

Example 2 Double diluting a drug e.g. sodium bicarbonate
A dose of 1.5 ml is needed, so double dilute with WFI to 3 ml total in syringe
However, you will 'lose' much of this syringe volume within
the line during priming
Tip: So, draw up double of everything in 1 syringe i.e. 3 ml of sodium bicarbonate and 3 ml WFI and run through the IV line until 3 ml is left in the syringe

The above principles can be applied to any drug that needs further dilution to administer it

---

Box 2.24b   Administering drugs when you need to give very small amounts – FLOW CHART

Example: Ranitidine (preparation is 50 ml in 2 ml = 25 mg in 1 ml)
1 mg prescribed, so 0.04 ml is required, which is a very small quantity
to work with
Therefore, take out 1 ml (= 25 mg) from the drug vial

▽

Add to 4 ml of saline or WFI

▽

This makes 25 mg in 5 ml (5 mg in 1 ml)

▽

Work out your dose (1 mg) from this solution to enable you to give a greater
volume
New volume after dilution = 0.2 ml, which is much easier to draw up
NB: you can alter the volume that the drug is diluted into as long as you
always use the standard drug formula from Box 2.22 to work out how much
you need to draw up finally

**The above principles can be applied to any drug where you need to
draw up a larger volume to administer it safely**

Box 2.24c   Making drugs more concentrated for infusion – FLOW CHART

To make a drug infusion more concentrated in volume restricted neonates, a
larger initial dose of the drug is added to the syringe in the first instance
in the same volume e.g. double the drug amount will give the desired
dose in half the volume
The formula in Box 2.23 is then used in the same way
In other words, adding more drug gives the same dose but in a smaller
volume

**The above principle can be applied to any drug infusion where
you need to restrict volume but keep the drug dosage
the same**

 Check local guidance on agreed strategies for drug administration

---

	Stop and think		**Standard precautions**
	Local variations		**Signposts**

Always apply standard precautions when drawing up and administering any drug by any route.

The space below can be used to record any local variations and practice points specific to your own unit.

Drugs and drug administration: Glossary

Catheter: A small, thin plastic tube through which fluids are given.

Central line: An IV line inserted into a vein, often in the arm, and threaded from there into a larger vein in the body close to the heart. Used to deliver drugs or IV solutions that would be irritating to smaller veins.

Contraindication: A condition which makes a particular treatment or procedure potentially inadvisable.

Half-life: The time taken for a therapeutic drug level to fall to half its original value.

Intradermal: Within the layers of the skin.

Intramuscular: Within the muscle.

Intravenous: Through a vein.

Parenteral: Route other than via the mouth and digestive tract.

Peak: Therapeutic level of a drug at its highest.

Peripheral line: An IV cannula inserted into a peripheral vein.

Subcutaneous: Applied under the skin.

Therapeutic: The dose of a drug needed to treat a disease or obtain the desired response.

Toxicity: Harmful effects of a drug at high levels.

Trough: The lowest level at which a medicine is present in the body.

> The Glossary for *Fluid balance and electrolytes* is also relevant for this topic.

Drug and drug administration: References

Blair, K. (2011). *Medicines Management in Children's Nursing*. Exeter: Learning Matters.

NMC (2010). Standards for Medicines Management. http://www.nmc-uk.org/Documents/NMC-Publications/NMC-Standards-for-medicines-management.pdf

Sammons, H., & Conroy, S. (2008). How do we ensure safe prescribing for children?. *Archives of Disease in Childhood*, 93(2), 98–99.

Developmental care in the neonatal unit

The second part of this chapter addresses the principles of developmental care in the neonatal unit. This is an area concerned with promoting the well-being of the neonate by the application of developmentally supportive measures (Symington and Pinelli, 2006) and promoting an environment that minimizes stress and disturbance. Developmental care involves many important concepts aimed at optimizing the neonate's outcome. Appropriate positioning of the neo-nate serves as a specific example of how care can be developmentally supportive. The aim is to position the neonate appropriately and comfortably, while supporting their limbs and head, to avoid any short- or long-term effects to the skin or muscular system. (Balaguer et al., 2013; Madlinger-Lewis et al., 2014; Pineda et al., 2014). In addition, *gentle handling* emphasizes the need to treat the neonate with care according to their behavioural and physiological cues, an important principle of cue-based care (Kalyn et al., 2003; Pinelli and Symington, 2005; Mörelios et al., 2006; Pickler et al., 2013).

Figure 2.15 and Boxes 2.25 and 2.26 address these three elements of developmental care; an overview of the concept, principles of good positioning and recognizing and minimizing stress. The role of the parents is an integral part of this area of care.

Related topics: see also *Environmental care, Psychosocial care of the family* and *Pain management*. These areas are closely related to optimizing the comfort, well-being and outcomes of neonates within a family perspective.

Developmental care should be part of the holistic management strategy, particularly of the preterm neonate, however sick. Individualized programmes should be tailored to their specific needs (Haumont et al., 2013; Pickler et al., 2013).

Figure 2.15 Developmental Care principles – DIAGRAM

Parental involvement
Parents should be involved in interventions to help promote understanding of neonate's behavioural cues and practice of cue-based care

Minimize painful procedures
Provide appropriate pain relief and comforting techniques to reduce stress. Non-nutritive sucking, containment, gentle holding, hands together, grasping a finger

Support of behavioural organization
Maintain a balance between autonomic, physiological, motor, attention/interaction and self-regulation (consoling)

Developmental care
Create an environment that minimizes stress while providing developmentally appropriate care for the neonate and family

Control environment
Minimize the neonate's exposure to noxious stimuli such as strong fragrances, open alcohol swabs and clinical procedures

Optimal handling
To minimize stress and uncontrolled responses. Keep in a flexed and contained position. Move neonate slowly and keep them in contact with the supporting surface. Introduce touch slowly and allow time for the neonate to respond and adjust

Cue-based care
In response to the neonate's behavioural cues, provide and modifiy sensory stimulation, cue-based feeding to pace feeds, time out during care procedures

 Check local guidance on developmental care policy

Box 2.25   Positioning the neonate – CHECKLIST

Neonates should be positioned with:
- symmetrical postures
- flexion of limbs
- shoulder and hip flexion and adduction
- hands near face
- neutral alignment of ankles and hips
- neutral alignment of head and neck whenever possible
- the use of swaddling or nesting to provide boundaries (Figures 2.16–2.18).

(continued)

Figure 2.16 Side-lying

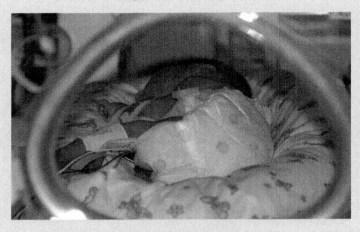

Figure 2.17 Prone

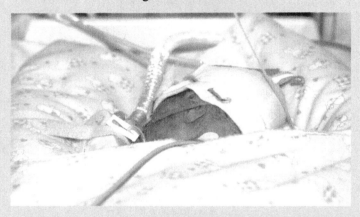

Figure 2.18 Supine

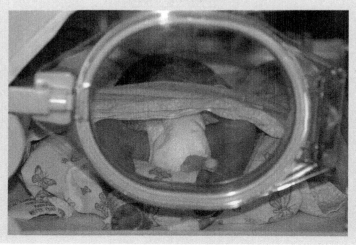

Once a sick neonate's condition has improved in special or transitional care prior to discharge, remember to always place the neonate supine, as per the guidelines for the prevention of sudden infant death syndrome (SIDS).

Box 2.26   Neonatal stress cues and interventions – CHECKLIST

Stress cues	Interventions
Autonomic signs • Colour changes • Changes in vital signs • Visceral responses (vomiting, gagging, hiccups) • Sneezing • Yawning	• Grouping care activities and appropriate timing of care in line with 'minimal handling' • Individualizing care to the cues of each neonate. When possible, slow the pace of what you are doing or give the neonate a break, if signs of stress are noted • Use of appropriate supported positioning. Use of rolls and other supports to help keep the neonate in a comfortable flexed position
Motor signs Flailing movements Finger splaying (holding fingers spread wide apart) Hyperextension of arms or legs **Behaviours** Diffuse sleep states (twitching, grimacing, not resting peacefully) Glassy-eyed ('tuning out') Gaze aversion Staring Panicked look Irritability (hard to console)	• Wrapping/containment • Tactile soothing/skin to skin • Breast-feeding/breast milk • Looking at and listening to the immediate environment from the neonate's perspective and decreasing environmental sensors • Holding a neonate's hand (gently placing a finger in the palm, which stimulates the grasp reflex) • Pacifier/sucking • Encouraging self-regulatory behaviours – these include changing position, hand-to-mouth, grasping, sucking and hand clasping • Self-regulatory behaviours will be seen more often as the neonate gets closer to 40 weeks' gestation

☛ Also refer to *Pain management*

◉ Check local guidance

Recognition of behavioural cues during periods of handling informs carers when neonates become stressed. Even the most basic of care procedures can cause physiological stress (Wang and Chang, 2004; Catelin et al., 2005; Lyngstad et al., 2014) and therefore a 'time-out' period should be initiated.

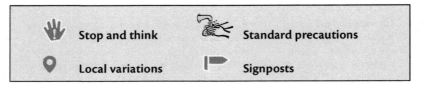

Stop and think   Standard precautions

Local variations   Signposts

Always observe thorough hand washing when handling or re-positioning neonates.

The space below can be used to record any local variations and practice points specific to your own unit.

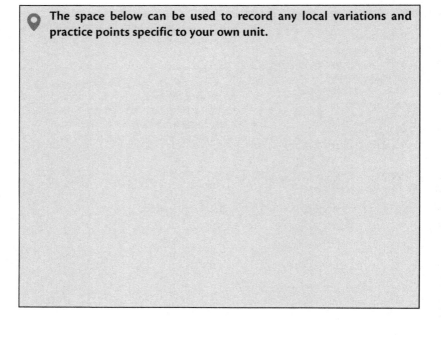

Developmental care: Glossary

Behavioural organization: A term used to describe the establishment of integration between a neonates' physiological and behavioural states. Can also be termed 'state regulation'.

Behavioural states: The behaviours exhibited by a neonate, namely deep sleep, light sleep, fussy, awake and alert, crying.

Cue-based care: Supportive care initiated in response to the neonates' behavioural cues or signs.

Developmental care: An approach to caring for premature neonates that places an emphasis on their individual needs, recognizing their behavioural cues and working with the family to minimize stress and optimize developmental outcomes.

NIDCAP: Neonatal Individualized Developmental Care and Assessment Program. A formal programme of developmental care requiring training.

Time out: Allowing a period of rest when a neonate exhibits signs of stress to allow them to calm and stabilize.

<blockquote>
The Glossaries for *Environmental care* and *Pain management* are also relevant for this topic and provide further terminology.
</blockquote>

Developmental care: References

Balaguer, A., Escribano, J., Roqué, I., Figuls, M., and Rivas-Fernandez, M. (2013). Infant position in neonates receiving mechanical ventilation. *Cochrane Database of Systematic Reviews*, Issue 3. Art. No.: CD003668.

Catelin, C., Tordjman, S., Morin, V., Oger, E., and Sizun, J. (2005). Clinical, physiologic, and biologic impact of environmental and behavioral interventions in neonates during a routine nursing procedure. *The Journal of Pain*. 6 (12): 791–797.

Haumont, D., Amiel-Tison, C., Casper, C., Conneman, N., Ferrari, F., Huppi, P., and Westrup, B. (2013). NIDCAP and developmental care: A European perspective. *Pediatrics*. 132 (2): e551–e552.

Kalyn, A., Blatz, S., Feuerstake, S., Paes, B., and Bautista, C. (2003). Closed suctioning of intubated neonates maintains better physiologic stability: A randomized trial. *Journal of Perinatology*. 23 (3): 218–222.

Lyngstad, L.T., Tandberg, B.S., Storm, H., Ekeberg, B.L., and Moen, A. (2014). Does skin-to-skin contact reduce stress during diaper change in preterm infants? *Early Human Development*. 90 (4): 169–172.

Madlinger-Lewis, L., Reynolds, L., Zarem, C., Crapnell, T., Inder, T., and Pineda, R. (2014). The effects of alternative positioning on preterm infants in the neonatal intensive care unit:

A randomized clinical trial. *Research in Developmental Disabilities*. 35 (2): 490–497.

Mörelius, E., Hellström-Westas, L., Carlén, C., Norman, E., and Nelson, N. (2006). Is a nappy change stressful to neonates? *Early Human Development*. 82 (10): 669–676.

Pickler, R.H., McGrath, J.M., Reyna, B.A., Tubbs-Cooley, H.L., Best A., M., Lewis, M., Cone, S., and Wetzel, P.A. (2013). Effects of the neonatal intensive care unit environment on preterm infant oral feeding. *Research and Reports in Neonatology*. 3: 15–20.

Pineda, R.G., Neil, J., Dierker, D., Smyser, C.D., Wallendorf, M., Kidokoro, H., and Inder, T. (2014). Alterations in brain structure and neurodevelopmental outcome in preterm infants hospitalized in different neonatal intensive care unit environments. *The Journal of Pediatrics*. 164 (1): 52–60.

Pinelli, J., and Symington, A.J. (2005). Non-nutritive sucking for promoting physiologic stability and nutrition in preterm infants. *Cochrane Database of Systematic Reviews*. Issue 4. Art. No.: CD001071.

Symington, A.J., and Pinelli, J. (2006). Developmental care for promoting development and preventing morbidity in preterm infants. Cochrane Database of Systematic Reviews. Issue 2. Art. No.: CD001814.

Wang, Y.W., and Chang, Y.J. (2004). A preliminary study of bottom care effects on premature infants' heart rate and oxygen saturation. *Journal of Nursing Research*. 12 (2): 161–168.

Further reading: Developmental care

A sound body of theory underpins this topic and the reader may refer to the following selected open access resources to explore further.

Armstrong, E.K., Ball, A.L., and Leatherbarrow, J. (2012). Constructing a programme of change to improve the provision of family-centred developmental care on a neonatal unit. *Infant*. 8 (3): 86–90. http://www.infantgrapevine.co.uk/pdf/inf_045_han.pdf

Goldstein, R. (2012). Developmental care for premature infants: A state of mind. *Pediatrics*. 129 (5): e1322–e1323. http://pediatrics.aappublications.org/content/129/5/e1322.full

Kleberg, A. (2006). *Promoting preterm infants' development and mother-child interaction: Neonatal individualized developmental care and assessment programme (NIDCAP)*. http://diss.kib.ki.se/2006/91-7140-850-9/thesis.pdf

LaRossa, M.M. (2014). *Understanding preterm infant behavior in the NICU*. http://www.pediatrics.emory.edu/divisions/neonatology/dpc/nicubeh.html

Environmental care

This unit follows on appropriately from the preceding one as it turns now to environmental care.

Environmental care includes management of the surroundings within the neonatal unit, incorporating the acoustic, light and thermal environment. The potentially harmful effects of the external surroundings on the preterm neonate are well documented (White, 2006; Lasky and Williams, 2009; Peng et al., 2013). The following unit addresses the concept of environmental care with an overview of practice points to optimize the neonatal environment (Figure 2.20).

> Related topics: see also *Developmental care* as environmental care is an important part of this as a whole. In addition, *Thermal care* provides further information on the importance of managing the thermal environment specifically.

Figure 2.19 Incubator with cover

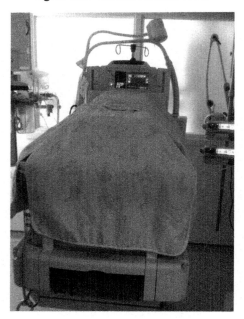

Figure 2.20 Optimizing the neonatal unit environment – DIAGRAM

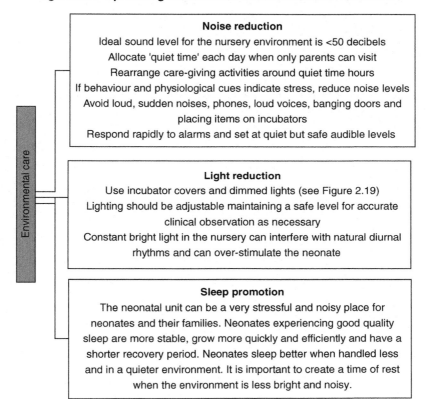

Environmental care

Noise reduction
Ideal sound level for the nursery environment is <50 decibels
Allocate 'quiet time' each day when only parents can visit
Rearrange care-giving activities around quiet time hours
If behaviour and physiological cues indicate stress, reduce noise levels
Avoid loud, sudden noises, phones, loud voices, banging doors and placing items on incubators
Respond rapidly to alarms and set at quiet but safe audible levels

Light reduction
Use incubator covers and dimmed lights (see Figure 2.19)
Lighting should be adjustable maintaining a safe level for accurate clinical observation as necessary
Constant bright light in the nursery can interfere with natural diurnal rhythms and can over-stimulate the neonate

Sleep promotion
The neonatal unit can be a very stressful and noisy place for neonates and their families. Neonates experiencing good quality sleep are more stable, grow more quickly and efficiently and have a shorter recovery period. Neonates sleep better when handled less and in a quieter environment. It is important to create a time of rest when the environment is less bright and noisy.

 Check local guidance

References: Raoof and Ohlsson (2013); Szymczak and Shellhaas (2014); Morag and Ohlsson (2013)

    Exposure to inappropriate noise levels may cause physiological instability, agitation and disrupted sleep patterns. The aim of environmental care therefore, is to mimic the uterine environment, promote physical stability, avoid hypoxia and support organized sleep patterns and circadian rhythms (Peng et al., 2013).

 Stop and think   **Standard precautions**

 Local variations   **Signposts**

Always observe thorough hand washing practices when handling the neonate and ensure the immediate neonatal environment is kept clean.

The space below can be used to record any local variations and practice points specific to your own unit.

Environmental care: Glossary

Decibel: A unit used to measure the intensity of a sound.

Environment: The surroundings or conditions in which a neonate is nursed. Comprises light and noise levels, extent and frequency of disruption and the thermal milieu.

Minimal handling: Ensuring disturbances to the neonate are kept to a minimum and care interventions are performed only if necessary, recognising and attending to behavioural cues at all times. Links closely with Developmental care.

Quiet time: A designated period of calm and tranquillity without any disturbance to the neonate to enable them to settle, sleep and resume state regulation.

> The Glossaries for *Developmental care* and *Thermal care* are also relevant for this topic.

Environmental care: References

Lasky, R.E. and Williams, A.L. (2009). Noise and light exposures for extremely low birth weight newborns during their stay in the neonatal intensive care unit. *Pediatrics.* 123: 540.

Morag, I. and Ohlsson, A. (2013). Cycled light in the intensive care unit for preterm and low birth weight infants. *Cochrane Database of Systematic Reviews.* Issue 8. Art. No.: CD006982.

Peng, N.H., Bachman, J., Jenkins, R., Chen, C.H., Chang, Y.C., Chang, Y.S., and Wang, T.M. (2013). Relationships between environmental stressors and stress biobehavioral responses of preterm infants in NICU. *Advances in Neonatal Care.* 13: S2-S10.

Raoof, A. and Ohlsson, A. (2013). Noise reduction management in the neonatal intensive care unit for preterm or very low birthweight infants (Protocol). *Cochrane Database of Systematic Reviews.* Issue 1. Art. No.: CD010333.

Szymczak, S.E. and Shellhaas, R.A. (2014). Impact of NICU design on environmental noise. *Journal of Neonatal Nursing.* 20 (2): 77–81.

White, R. (2006). Recommended standards for newborn ICU design. *J Perinatol.* 26: S2–S18.

Fluid balance and electrolytes

This unit focuses on the management of fluid and electrolyte therapy.

This is an important area because most neonates in the neonatal unit require intravenous (IV) fluids at some point and experience shifts of fluids between intracellular, extracellular and vascular compartments (Ambalavanan, 2014). Therefore, careful attention to fluid and electrolyte balance is required as serious morbidity may result from imbalances.

In this unit, guidance follows on calculating fluids, electrolytes and daily allowances (Boxes 2.27a and 2.27b), administering electrolytes (Box 2.28) and IV infusion care (Box 2.29 and Table 2.19).

Related topics: see also *Drugs* for relevant formulas and *Gastrointestinal care and feeding* for guidance on enteral feeding and TPN. *Renal care* outlines the principles of fluid output.

Optimum fluid management is about ensuring a balance between input and output. However, it is not always straightforward in a sick and/or preterm neonate who may be compromised and immature (Hartnoll, 2003; Modi, 2004; Bell and Acarregui, 2008).

Box 2.27a   Calculating fluids and daily allowances – CHECKLIST

- As a general guide, neonates admitted to NNU should receive quantities of fluids per day calculated according to their birth weight until this has been regained, then calculations are based on current weight.
- Total volumes of fluid include all infusions and/or enteral feeds, but do not usually include bolus drugs or intravascular volume.

The following table is an example of a basic fluid regimen (days refer to periods of 24 hours after birth).
Multiply the required volume per day by the weight and divide by 24 hours to obtain the hourly input.

(continued)

	Day 1	Day 2	Day 3	Day 4	Day 5	Day 6	Day 7	
All premature infants	60	90	120	120	150	180	180	ml/kg/day
Term infants	50	70	90	110	130	150	150	ml/kg/day

Exceptions: Neonates with a low blood glucose may need their fluid allowance increasing to enable them to receive more glucose. Conversely, a neonate born with hypoxia may require restricted fluids to avoid circulatory overload from compromised kidneys; their fluid allowance is therefore decreased from the usual expected intake.

- Weight is an important parameter for fluid requirement assessment. Expect 5–10% weight loss from birth weight (BW), before weight is regained
- Balance can be a challenge between dehydration and overload (remember inappropriate anti-diuretic hormone (ADH))
- Neonates receiving IV fluids may have weight and serum electrolytes measured daily
- Monitor output – urine output should be a minimum of 1ml/kg/day on Day 1, then 2–3 ml/kg/day thereafter. Weigh nappies (1 g = 1 ml urine)
- Fluid balance along with weight are important to make decisions about liberalizing/increasing fluids

  The most important point is to tailor fluids to individual needs

📍 Check local guidance on fluid regimens as variations may apply

Source: Adapted with kind permission from Bart's Health Neonatal Unit, Royal London NHS Trust, London

---

Box 2.27b   Glucose and electrolyte requirements – CHECKLIST

- *Glucose:* On day 1, 10% dextrose. Higher concentrations may be required if hypoglycaemic

Electrolyte intake is varied according to plasma values but the following is a guide:

- *Calcium:* In extremely premature infants, calcium may be needed on the first day of life (start at 1 mmol/kg/day)
- *Sodium:* Needed once the neonate develops a natriuresis (as evidenced by increased urine output, falling weight and sometimes falling serum sodium)

(continued)

Amounts needed may vary between 2–4 mmol/kg/day baseline, up to 10 mmol/kg/day in preterm neonates with large urinary losses
- *Potassium:* Should not normally be given on the first day of life. Should only be started once there is good urine output, serum potassium <5 mmol/l and satisfactory creatinine. Start at 2–4 mmol/kg/day
- *Replacement of GI losses (surgical):* these should be replaced with normal saline with potassium added

📍   Check local guidance on electrolyte administration

References: Hartnoll (2003); Modi (2004); Bell and Acarregui (2008)

🖐   **Care must be taken when administering electrolytes intra-venously as they are *hypertonic* solutions potentially causing significant damage to the tissue if there is any extravasation. Observe the IV site very regularly.**

Box 2.28   Giving electrolytes – FLOW CHART

Adding electrolytes to an infusion bag of maintenance

To work out how many mmols should be added to infusion/maintenance fluids to give a required dose of electrolytes:

Example 1: For maintenance with no enteral feed or other infusions

$$\frac{500 \text{ ml (bags volume)}}{\text{Total maintenance volume (ml) to be given in 24 hours}^{**}} \times \text{mmol/kg/day} \times \text{weight}$$

Example = **1.5 kg neonate on 90 ml/kg/day needing 3 mmol/kg/day of sodium**

$$\frac{500}{135} \times 3 \times 1.5 \text{ kg} = 16.6 \text{ mmol of sodium to be added}$$

** Total volume to be given in 24 hours refers to the maintenance volume required by the neonate as total ml. In this first example, this is 1.5 × 90 = 135 ml. If the neonate is on drug infusions and/or feeds that are included (i.e. not extra) then the total volume should have the volume of drug infusions/feed subtracted. This is illustrated in the example overleaf

(continued)

Example 2: For maintenance fluid with multiple infusions

$$\frac{500\ ml}{\text{total maintenance volume (ml) to be given in 24 hours **}} \times \text{mmol/kg/day} \times \text{weight}$$

Example =
Total fluid is 120 ml/kg/day. Weight is 3 kg
You want to give 2 mmol/kg/day of K+
Umbilical artery catheter (UAC) infusion is running at 1 ml/hour,
dopamine is running at 0.5 ml/hour and insulin at 0.3 ml/hour

Calculation:
120 ml **x** 3 (kg) in 24 hours
= 360 ml
= 15 ml/hour
Infusions are 1.8 ml/hour
15−1.8 = 13.2 ml/hour
13.2 x 24
= 316.8 ml

$$\frac{500}{316.8} \times 2 \times 3\ kg$$

= 9.4 mmol of K+ to be added

To work out how many mmol/kg/day a baby is actually receiving …
The formula is reversed
i.e. for Example 1 previously **…**
16.6 mmol sodium has been added to 500 ml of maintenance and
the neonate is on 90ml/kg
How much sodium is the baby getting in mmol/kg/day?
16.6 divided by the weight divided by 500 ml
multiplied by 135 gives you 3 mmol/kg/day

Check local guidance

Electrolytes should be prescribed and administered according to individual need and evaluated on a regular basis.

IV infusion care

The importance of vigilance with IV devices and assessment must be emphasized to prevent both infection and damage to veins and IV sites, particularly in relation to the fragile vascular system in the neonatal population (Douglas et al., 2009; Dioni et al., 2014). For long-term IV infusions, the use of a percutaneous inserted central catheter (PICC) is commonplace (Ainsworth et al., 2007). However, peripheral venous cannulas need to be used frequently for drugs and so risk prevention is essential. Two frameworks can be applied to this: the IV care bundle (Box 2.29) and the visual infusion phlebitis score (VIPS) IV site assessment tool (Table 2.19).

Box 2.29   Intravenous infusion care bundle – CHECKLIST

- Hand washing
- Assess need for IV cannula/PICC line
- Site inspection hourly and document
- Use VIPS tool (see Table 2.19 overleaf) and document
- If lines are not required, remove
- Access – use aseptic non-touch technique (ANTT)
- Clean all ports with alcohol swab and allow to dry
- Administration set replacement – depends on local policy and the solution being administered (e.g. TPN; 24–48 hours, IV fluids with additives; 24 hours)

Standard precautions are an integral component of this area of practice to prevent cross infection.

Check local guidance on agreed procedure on IV site care and changing lines

Reference: UK Department of Health (2007)

Care bundles consist of key clinical procedures which, when performed together, help to reduce the risk of infection (Maki, 2008; RCN, 2010).

Table 2.19   Visual infusion phlebitis scale (VIPS) – SUMMARY TABLE

Appearance	Score	Stage of Phlebitis
IV site appears healthy	0	No signs
Action: observe cannula		
One of the following signs is evident	1	First signs
• Slight pain near IV site or • Slight redness near IV site Action: observe cannula		
Two of the following are evident	2	Early stage
• Pain at IV site • Redness • Swelling Action: re-site cannula		
All of the following signs are evident	3	Medium stage
• Pain along path of cannula • Redness around site • Swelling Action: re-site cannula and consider treatment		
All of the following signs are evident/ extensive	4	Start of advanced stage
• Pain along path of cannula • Redness around site • Swelling • Action: re-site cannula and consider treatment		
All of the following signs are extensive	5	Advanced stage
• Pain along path of cannula • Redness around site and swelling • Extravasation Action: initiate treatment/re-site cannula		
*Treatment: stop infusion, remove IV device, elevate limb, apply comfort measures. For peripheral site extravasation injury, follow local policy and consider subcutaneous irrigation with normal saline (with or without hyaluronidase)		
Check local guidance on agreed procedure on IV site checking		

Source: Reprinted from Higginson, R and Parry, A., Phlebitis: Treatment, care and prevention. Nursing Times. (2011). 107/36. Pages 18–21, with permission from Emap Ltd (original source: Jackson A (1998) Infection control: a battle in vein infusion phlebitis. Nursing Times; 94/4, 68–71)

Extravasation injury can arise rapidly if administering hypertonic drugs, glucose or electrolyte concentrations (Wilkins and Emmerson, 2004). All intravenous devices/sites should be assessed regularly and documented.

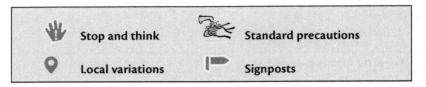

Stop and think   Standard precautions

Local variations   Signposts

Always apply standard precautions with any clinical practice involving accessing the venous or arterial system invasively.

The space below can be used to record any local variations and practice points specific to your own unit.

Fluid balance: Glossary

Aseptic non-touch technique (ANTT): See Infection and immunisations.

Dehydration: Fluid depleted as exhibited by sunken fontanelles and eyes, dry, poor skin turgor, thready pulses, low urine output (oliguria) and high specific gravity on urinalysis.

Diuresis: Increased production of urine.

Electrolytes: A substance that ionizes when dissolved in suitable solvents such as water (e.g. sodium, potassium, magnesium, calcium).

Extravasation: The leakage of intravenous drugs from the vein into the surrounding tissue.

Inappropriate anti-diuretic hormone (ADH): Excretion of ADH despite normal blood plasma volume, a condition which can be seen in preterm neonates with respiratory distress syndrome who are ventilated, leading to more water than is actually required being reabsorbed from the kidneys back into the blood stream.

Maintenance: Daily fluid requirement.

Natriuresis: Excretion of sodium in the urine.

Oedema: An excess of fluid in the cavities or tissues of the body.

Overload: The state of having too much fluid within the body.

PICC (percutaneous inserted central catheter) line: A type of central line, which is placed in one of the major blood vessels. Also known as a 'long line'. (Percutaneous catheters are distinct from Hickman® and Broviac® lines that are surgically inserted, skin tunnelled central lines more commonly seen in surgical units).

Visual infusion phlebitis score (VIPS): A tool for monitoring intravenous infusion sites and determining when access should be removed.

> The Glossaries for *Drugs, Gastrointestinal care and feeding* and *Renal care* are also relevant for this topic.

Fluid balance: References

Ainsworth, S., Clerihew, L., and McGuire, W. (2007). Percutaneous central venous catheters versus peripheral cannulae for delivery of parenteral nutrition in neonates. *Cochrane Database of Systematic Reviews.* Issue 3. Art. No.: CD004219.

Ambalavanan, N. (2014). Fluid, electrolyte, and nutrition management of the newborn. http://emedicine.medscape.com/article/976386-overview

Bell, E.F. and Acarregui, M.J. (2008). Restricted versus liberal water intake for preventing morbidity and mortality in preterm infants. *Cochrane Database of Systematic Reviews.* Issue 1. Art. No.: CD000503. DOI: 10.1002/14651858.CD000503.pub2.

Dioni, E., Franceschini, R., Marzollo, R., Oprandi, D., and Chirico, G. (2014). Central vascular catheters and infections. *Early Human Development.* 90: S51–S53.

Douglas, L., Aspin, A., Jimmeson, N., and Lawrance, V. (2009). Central venous access devices; review of practice. *Paediatric Nursing.* 2 (5): 19–22.

Hartnoll, G. (2003). Basic principles and practical steps in the management of fluid balance in the newborn. *Seminars in Neonatology.* 8: 307–313.

Higginson, R. and Parry, A. (2011). Phlebitis: Treatment, care and prevention. *Nursing Times.* 107: 36 18–21.

Maki, D.G. (2008). Improving the safety of peripheral intravenous catheters. *BMJ.* 337 (7662): 122–123.

Modi, N. (2004). Management of fluid balance in the very immature neonate. *Arch Dis Child.* 89: F108–111.

Royal College of Nursing (2010). *Standards for infusion therapy.* London: RCN.

UK Department of Health (2007). *High impact intervention No 2; Peripheral intravenous cannula care bundle.* London: DH.

Wilkins, C.E. and Emmerson, A.J.B. (2004). Extravasation injuries on neonatal units. *Archives of Diseases in Childhood. Fetal and Neonatal Edition.* 89 (3): F274–275.

Gastrointestinal care and feeding

This chapter covers the topic of neonatal feeding and related topics.

A healthy neonate will feed on demand via either breast or bottle without problems. However, in neonatal care, feeding management and support is often necessary for sick and immature neonates. Establishing postnatal nutrition and assessing the gastrointestinal tract (GIT) are essential components of neonatal care (King, 2005) and are covered in Figure 2.21, Tables 2.20 and 2.21, and Boxes 2.30–2.35.

Related topics: see *Fluid balance and electrolytes* as enteral and fluid volumes need to be considered together. *Weight* is also important in relation to the monitoring of adequate nutrition and weight gain. In addition, see *Surgical* chapter to link with important practice areas relating to gastrointestinal tract (GIT) surgery and conditions.

Figure 2.21 Overview of feeding methods – FLOW CHART

Intensive care
- Intravenous (IV) fluids (dextrose) from birth
- Total parenteral nutrition (TPN) thereafter
- Start enteral nutrition as early as possible as tolerated
- Trophic feeding (minimal enteral nutrition) is extra to IV volumes using breast milk. See Box 2.33a

High dependency
- Enteral feeding via nasogastric/orogastric tube (NGT/OGT)
- TPN continues and is weaned as enteral feeding is increased, as tolerated.
- NGT/OGT feeding is usually given as bolus (gavage). Continuous feeding may carried out in cases of severe reflux.
- Other forms of feeding may also be needed for surgical reasons; e.g. gastrostomy, short gut.
- Breast milk is preferable to formula if possible. See Box 2.33b

Special care
- When ready, start the transition from tube to oral feeding
- The ideal method is breast feeding with support from a feeding specialist if available, in line with UNICEF (2013) Baby Friendly guidelines.
- Preterm neonates receive supplementation via breast fortifier or enteral daily doses of vitamins, iron and folic acid.
- If formula fed, special formulas are used as appropriate for neonate's gestation, weight and nutritional status

 Check local guidance

The aim is always to feed a neonate *as early as possible* as long as their physiological condition, gestation and ability to tolerate enteral feeding allows.

Table 2.20   Nutritional requirements in the neonate – SUMMARY TABLE

A neonate requires the following for adequate growth

Carbohydrate (energy)* Protein*
Optimum Energy: Protein ratio* (See below*)
Lipids – long chain polyunsaturated fatty acids

Vitamins
Thiamin, Riboflavin, Niacin, Vitamin B12, Folate, Vitamin C,
Vitamin A, Vitamin D

Minerals
Calcium, phosphorus, magnesium, sodium, potassium, chloride, iron, zinc, copper,
selenium and iodine

Supplementation
Supplementation of breast milk by fortifier adds protein and energy and is often
required in the preterm neonate when they are on full feeds and TPN has
been discontinued.
Vitamins, folic acid, iron, sodium and phosphate are required if milk is unfortified.
(*References*: Kuschel and Harding, 2004; Embleton, 2013)

Recommendations (ESPGHAN)

*Nutrient	Term	Preterm
Energy kcal/kg/day	96–120	110–135
Protein g/kg/day	2.1	3.4–4.2 <1 kg 4–4.5
Energy: Protein ratio	1–1.8 kg 3.2–3.6g/100kcal (12.8–14.4%) <1 kg 3.6–4.1g/100kcal (14.4–16.4%)	

Check local guidance on feeding regimens and specific advice

Any specific nutritional advice should be discussed with the neonatal dietician as an important member of the multi-disciplinary team.

Handling and preparing expressed breast milk

As seen above, the ideal milk for any neonate, particularly those born preterm and/or small, is breast milk and this is consistently recommended to be the default choice of enteral nutrition in and out of hospital (Henderson et al., 2007). However, for sick neonates who have spent much time in the neonatal unit, breast-feeding is not possible for some considerable time and so a mother should be encouraged to express her milk (UNICEF, 2013; Nyquist et al., 2013). In addition, of course, not all mothers continue to produce milk for varying reasons or she may choose to feed using formula preparations when discharged home; hence, formula milks are used. Boxes 2.30 and 2.31 address the making up of breast milk preparation and powdered formula milk, respectively.

> **Another important member of the multi-disciplinary team is the feeding specialist or someone allocated to supporting and advising on feeding, for both staff and parents. Advice includes how to prepare and store breastmilk for feeding.**

Box 2.30   Handling and storage of expressed breast milk – FLOW CHART

Expressing

- All mothers in the hospital setting should be taught how to express, label and store their milk in line with the local Trust standard
- The expressed breast milk (EBM) for each neonate should have a designated space in the fridge
- Tips for mother: start expressing within 6 hours from delivery, express at least once between midnight and 6am, hand pumping is useful to collect colostrum followed by electric pump and express 8–10 times per 24 hour period until milk supply is established, avoiding long gaps of more than 6 hours (East of England Perinatal Network (EEPN), 2012)

▽

Making up feeds

- In line with local policy and using standard precautions to prevent infection, feeds should be made up in sterile syringes or bottles to suit the desired qualities and feeding pattern for each neonate. Fortifier may be added

▽

Labelling

- Labelling should include neonate's hospital number, name, date and time milk was expressed/defrosted

(continued)

▽
Storage
- Milk should be used within recommended timescales. A guide is to use milk within 4 hours at room temperature, any milk defrosted and storied in the fridge to be used within 24 hours and to freeze breast milk for no longer than 3 months (hospital).

▽
- Unused breast milk should be discarded if not used within these time periods
- The fridge temperature should be 2°C −4°C and freezer −20°C
- Never refreeze milk, as this may increase the risk of bacterial growth
- Unused frozen expressed breast milk must be discarded after 3 months
- This guide is based on hospital-based care. Guidelines for home storage differ:
  o At home, breast milk can be stored in a sterilized container: in the fridge for up to 5 days at 4°C or lower, for 2 weeks in the ice compartment of a fridge and for up to 6 months in a freezer
  o Parents storing milk in their fridge at home should store it towards the back and not in the fridge door, to maintain a cooler temperature

▽
Defrosting
- Frozen milk should be thawed in the fridge
- Use milk within 24 hours after the start of the defrosting process

▽
Administration
- Remove a maximum of 4 hours worth of milk from the fridge
- Milk should be used in the order that it was expressed for the first 14 days to ensure baby gets all of the colostrum
- After 14 days, use the freshest milk available, and fresh milk in preference to frozen milk

 Strict infection control should be adhered to in relation to handling of any milk preparation.

Check local guidance on procedures for making up expressed breast milk and formula milk.

References: WHO (2007); UNICEF (2013); East of England Perinatal Network (EEPN) (2012)

Formula milk may be required if EBM supplies exhaust and donor milk is not available. In hospital, sterile pre-packed bottles are provided and the same rules apply to time left out at room temperature once opened. These are single use bottles, with any remaining milk being discarded once the desired volume has been given.

Box 2.31   Making up powdered formula milk – FLOW CHART

The aim is to ensure that when staff or parents make up powdered infant formula, it is prepared safely.

Points of note:
- Powdered infant formula is not a sterile product so if the feed is not prepared safely, bacteria can cause infection. Formula should be made up with water at a temperature of 70°C, which will kill these bacteria. It is recommended to make up a fresh bottle for each feed.

Making up a feed:
- Clean and disinfect the work surface, wash hands
- Use a sterile bottle   ▽
- Fill kettle with fresh tap water and allow to boil
- Allow kettle to cool for no longer than 30 minutes   ▽
- It is important that the water is still hot, 70°C, otherwise the bacteria in the milk powder may not be destroyed   ▽
- Pour the correct amount of water as per instructions into the sterile bottle   ▽
- Loosely fill the scoop and level it off using the leveller provided
- Add the number of scoops of milk powder as per instructions to the water
- Place lid on the bottle and shake the bottle until the powder is dissolved   ▽
- Always take care as the water is still hot enough to scald
- To cool milk, once powder is dissolved, hold the bottle under cold running water   ▽
- Place sterile teat onto bottle if to be used
- Test temperature of milk before giving it to the intended neonate
- Empty out the remaining water left in the kettle down the sink   ▽

Always ensure strict standard precautions are applied when making up formula milk

Along with the national guidance from the Department of Health, check local guidance on preparing milk for neonatal use.

References: NICE (2007); WHO (2007); UK Department of Health and Food Standards Agency (2011); National Health Service (2012); Royal College of Nursing (2013)

Total Parenteral Nutrition (TPN) and reducing TPN formulas

The aim of total parenteral nutrition (TPN) is to provide adequate nutrition to prevent catabolism and to promote growth, for those neonates who are unable to tolerate enteral feeds (Johnson, 2014) and for those in whom enteral feeding would constitute a risk. In some neonates, parenteral nutrition may supplement inadequate enteral intake, but for many it will constitute their only nutritional source (ElHassan and Kaiser, 2011). This unit provides an overview of TPN (Box 2.32a) including the formulas for when it is reduced/titrated once enteral feeding is increased (Box 2.32b).

> ✋ **TPN should be titrated/reduced as enteral feeding is advanced carefully according to the neonate's response and tolerance.**

Box 2.32a   Total parenteral nutrition (TPN) overview – SUMMARY TABLE

When?
- TPN is usually started within 24 hours of birth in neonates of ≤28 weeks gestation
- In older neonates, it is given following intestinal surgery or when enteral feeding is not possible

What?
- Parenteral nutrition should be introduced over a period of a few days, eventually providing balanced nutrition of carbohydrates, amino acids and lipids
- If urea levels are low, nitrogen (amino acid) may be increased; if growth is inadequate and there is no lipaemia, fat may be increased
- Supplementation with vitamins and trace elements will be provided, for example, magnesium and phosphate
- If there is persistent metabolic acidosis with a raised serum chloride, the neonate may be losing bicarbonate in the urine. In this case, acetate may be added in the TPN

Monitoring in TPN
- 4–6 hourly glucose until stable. Daily at least thereafter
- Daily urea and electrolyte measurement (including calcium)
- Regular albumin and phosphate estimations
- Regular weighing
- Regular monitoring for infection (Full blood count (FBC) and C reactive protein (CRP))
- Regular checks of serum bilirubin
- Weekly alkaline phosphatase and liver function tests (LFT)
- Daily urinalysis
- Observe for potential complications: line infection, thrombus and extravasation, hyperglycaemia, unconjugated hyperbilirubinaemia, cholestasis

Practice points:
Central line (e.g. percutaneously inserted central catheter (PICC) or 'long line' is necessary for TPN administration
Use of aseptic technique for care of central lines for TPN

(continued)

Break line as little as possible

TPN should not be not mixed with any drugs

Always use an infusion pump with a pressure alarm

If hyperglycaemic or glucose >1% in urine, insulin therapy may be required

 Strict infection control should be adhered to in relation to administering IV TPN. Use sterile giving sets and observe aseptic non-touch technique (ANTT) principles.

Check local guidance

Box 2.32b   Reducing TPN formulas – FLOW CHART

Calculation method of TPN rate adjustment

1) To obtain the rate of TPN/hour (TPN = Vamin + lipid)

Subtract hourly volume of feed and drug infusion from total volume of fluid/hour

2) To adjust the rate of Vamin/hour

$$\frac{(\text{Required TPN volume, obtained from above}) \times (\text{Prescribed rate of Vamin on the label})}{\text{Prescribed Rate of TPN (on the label)}}$$

3) To adjust the Rate of lipid/hour

$$\frac{(\text{Required TPN volume, obtained from above}) \times (\text{Prescribed rate of Lipid on the label})}{\text{Prescribed Rate of TPN (on the label)}}$$

Example 1:

Total fluid = 10 ml/hour

Feed = 4 ml/hour

Insulin = 1 ml/hour

Prescribed Vamin rate/hour on the label = 5.6 ml/hour

Prescribed lipid rate/hour on the label = 1.2 ml/hour

1) To obtain the rate of TPN/hour (TPN = Vamin + lipid)

$$10-4-1 = 5 \text{ ml}$$

2) To adjust the rate of Vamin/hour

$$\frac{5 \times 5.6}{(5.6 + 1.2)} = 4.1 \text{ ml}$$

(continued)

3) To adjust the rate of lipid/hour

$$\frac{5 \times 1.2}{(5.6 + 1.2)} = 0.88 = 0.9 \text{ ml}$$

Alternative method:

Find out the prescribed rates for Vamin and lipid (on the TPN bag)

Add the rates together = A

Work out the hourly rate that the neonate needs for their fluid requirement and subtract any drugs and milk. So …

The actual rate of fluids received (minus drugs/milk) = B

C = current rate for Vamin (before reduction)

D = current rate for lipid (before reduction)
So …

$$\frac{B \times C}{A}$$

This is the new rate for Vamin

And

$$\frac{B \times D}{A}$$

This is the new rate for lipid

Example 2:

1.7 kg baby on 120 ml/kg (= 8.5 ml/hour). On Vamin 7 and lipids 1.5
On milk of 1 ml/hour and has started morphine at 1 ml/hour
How to reduce the TPN accordingly and proportionally?

A Prescribed Vamin rate = 7 and prescribed lipid rate = 1.5
A = 7 + 1.5 = 8.5

B Neonate's hourly rate needed for fluid requirement minus any drug infusions and milk
= 8.5 minus 2 = 6.5

C Vamin rate = 7

D Lipid rate = 1.5

$$\frac{6.5 \times 7}{8.5} = 5.4 \text{ ml/hour as new Vamin rate}$$

(continued)

$$\frac{6.5 \times 1.5}{8.5} = 1.1 \text{ ml/hour as new lipid rate}$$

5.4 Vamin + 1.1 lipid + 2 ml (morphine and milk) = 8.5 ml/hour

Check local guidance for agreed formula to reduce/titrate TPN.

Source: Adapted with kind permission from Bart's Health Neonatal Unit, Royal London NHS Trust, London

Trophic feeding and advancement of feeds

The importance of early feeding should be emphasized for many reasons. However, for neonates unable to feed enterally, priming of the digestive tract by trophic feeding (minimal quantities) is necessary to encourage normal function (Morgan et al., 2013) and to prevent prolonged stasis of the bowel, which is associated with problems. Boxes 2.33a and 2.33b provide a guide for the commencement of trophic feeds and advancement thereafter followed by types of milk used in the neonatal unit.

> Minimal enteral nutrition or trophic feeding is *extra* to fluid requirements; when to include the volume should be carried out according to ongoing and regular assessment tailored to individual needs.

> **Box 2.33a   Advancing enteral feeds in the at-risk neonate – FLOW CHART**

Day 1 of feeding – Start enteral feeds as *trophic* feeds
Quantity of milk given, frequency and speed of feed advancement depends on whether the neonate is high, moderate or low risk
Advancing continues until full enteral volume is reached and TPN is reduced accordingly

East of England Perinatal Network (EEPN) (2012) refer to risk categories as:
High-risk neonate (<28 weeks gestation); <1 kg, unstable, hypoxic encephalopathy, small for gestational age, absent or reversed end diastolic flow antenatally, post necrotizing enterocolitis, polycythaemia, cardiac disease, certain drugs (steroids, indomethacin or ibuprofen)
Moderate-risk neonate (28 (+1 day) to 31 (+6 days) weeks gestation)
Standard-risk neonate (>32 weeks gestation)

Advance according to individual neonate and risk
For example
High risk – start with 2 hourly *trophic* feeds at 10–20 ml/kg/day and advance as indicated, for example, once or twice in 24 hours. Increase by 10 ml/kg/day no more than twice in 24 hours (as 1–2 hourly feeds) – aim for 180 ml/kg as tolerated/assessed

Moderate risk – start with 1–2 hourly feeds at 20 ml/kg/day and advance as indicated, for example, increase by 15 ml/kg/day no more than twice in 24 hours (as 1–2 hourly feeds) until full enteral volume is reached

Standard/low risk – start with 3 hourly feeds at 30–60 ml/kg/day and advance as indicated, for example, increase by 30 ml/kg/day as 3 hourly feeds until full enteral volume is reached

Individualized assessment is necessary. Exceptions always apply. Sub-groups e.g. <29 weeks and growth-restricted neonates may fail to tolerate even the above careful feeding regimen. A slower advancement of feeds may be required for these groups (Kempley et al., 2014).

🦐 Always ensure standard precautions are applied when handling milk for trophic feeds and thereafter.

📍 Check local guidance for agreed procedure for advancing enteral feeds.

Source: Adapted with kind permission from Nutrition Care Pathway, East of England Perinatal Network (EEPN, 2012)

Box 2.33b   Types of milk in neonatal care – FLOW CHART

- Breast milk is always the preferred choice of milk for any neonate of any gestation
- Term neonates who are healthy should feed on demand with support given as required for initiation and continuation of breast-feeding. If mother chooses not to breast feed, education and support should also be given in relation to safe administration of formula milk
- Expressed breast milk (EBM) is the first choice of milk for any preterm neonate
- For preterm neonates (<34 weeks gestation), breast milk fortifier can be added at an agreed time once they are able to tolerate 150 ml/kg/day
- If there is insufficient or no EBM, preterm formula can be used for neonates born <34 weeks gestation. Neonates >34 weeks can be given term formula as agreed by the neonatal team
- Donor breast milk (DBM) can be used where available, particularly if there is poor tolerance of formula milk
- Older preterm neonates (>34 weeks) can be breast-fed, given EBM or term formula if breast-feeding is not chosen or EBM is not available
- All the above decisions are subject to local policy and individualized assessment of weight gain and growth

📍 Check local guidance for agreed procedure for supplementation and choice of formula to use if applicable.

References: EEPN (2012); Leaf et al. (2012); Morgan et al. (2013)

🖐 **Full enteral feed volumes are subject to individual need and weight gain. If weight gain is adequate, a neonate can be fed on 150 ml/kg/day increasing to 180 ml/kg/day in cases where such gain is poor. This, however, may not be required if the neonate receives fortified EBM or preterm formula.**

Inserting and checking nasogastric and orogastric tubes

Gastric tube (gavage) feeding is commonplace within the neonatal unit. Therefore, it is essential that tubes are tested according to national guidance from the National Patient Safety Association (NPSA) (2005).

Box 2.34   Inserting and checking nasogastric and orogastric tubes – FLOW CHART

- An appropriately sized nasogastric or orogastric tube should be chosen e.g. 6 FG or 8 FG
- Markings enable accurate measurement of depth and length
- Aspirate stomach contents with a 10 ml syringe and test for an <u>acid</u> response using pH paper (Tho et al., 2011)
- Ensure you work through the NPSA (2005) flowchart and record all actions
- If there is no aspirate, the neonate can be repositioned
- pH should be 5.5 or less
- Consider factors that can contribute to a high gastric pH (6) such as the presence of amniotic fluid in a newborn, milk in the stomach, particularly if receiving 1–2 hourly feeds or use of medication to reduce stomach acid
- Once correct position of tube is ascertained, secure to face with approved method
- Check tube position using pH following initial tube insertion, before administering feeds or medication, following vomiting and if there is evidence of tube displacement (e.g. if tape is loose or visible tube appears longer or kinked)
- If on continuous feeds, synchronize tube checking with syringe changes

Always ensure standard precautions are applied when passing and checking feeding tubes.

Along with the national guidance from the NPSA (2005), check local guidance on care of nasogastric and orogastric tubes.

Measuring the correct length of nasogastric or orogastric tubes prior to passing is essential (Cirgin Ellett et al., 2012). Testing is carried out using pH paper and should not be done by the 'whoosh' test (auscultation of injected air entering the stomach) (NPSA, 2005).

Necrotizing enterocolitis assessment

Necrotizing enterocolitis (NEC) most commonly affects premature neonates and it is essential that anyone working in this field is mindful of the implications of this potentially devastating disease. The bowel becomes compromised when its blood supply is decreased before or following birth and bacteria that are normally present in the bowel invade the damaged area, causing more damage (Laukaityte, 2013). Prognosis is dependent on the amount of bowel affected and comorbidities (Schulzke et al., 2007). Vigilant assessment and supportive therapy is therefore essential (Gephart et al., 2012) and an example of a commonly cited approach for this is seen in Table 2.21. Finally Box 2.35 outlines the assessment of acute gastro-intestinal obstruction which is seen in NEC and other obstructive conditions.

> **Having a framework in which to assess a potentially devastating condition such as NEC assists in guiding appropriate management.**

Table 2.21 Necrotizing enterocolitis and Bells (modified) staging criteria – SUMMARY TABLE

Stage	Systemic signs	Abdominal signs	Signs on X-ray	Treatment
IA Suspected	Temperature instability, apnoea, bradycardia, lethargy	Gastric retention, abdominal distension, emesis, haem-positive stool	Normal or intestinal dilation, mild ileus	NBM, antibiotics
IB	Same as above	Bloody stool	Same as above	Same as IA
IIA Definite, mildly ill	Same as above	Same as above, plus absent bowel sounds with or without abdominal tenderness	Intestinal dilation, ileus, pneumatosis intestinalis	NBM, antibiotics for longer period than above

(continued)

Table 2.21   Continued

Stage	Systemic signs	Abdominal signs	Signs on X-ray	Treatment
IIB Definite, moderately ill	Same as above, plus mild metabolic acidosis and thrombocytopenia	Same as above, plus absent bowel sounds, definite tenderness	Same as IIA, plus ascites	NBM, antibiotics for longer period than above
IIIA Advanced, severely ill, intact bowel	Same as IIB, plus hypotension, bradycardia, severe apnoea, mixed acidosis, DIC and neutropenia	Same as above, plus signs of peritonitis, marked tenderness and abdominal distension	Same as IIA, plus ascites	NBM, antibiotics for at least 10 days, fluid resuscitation, inotropic support, ventilator therapy, paracentesis
IIIB Advanced, severely ill, perforated bowel	Same as IIIA	Same as IIIA	Same as above, plus pneumo-peritoneum	Same as IIA, plus surgery

Note: DIC: disseminated intravascular coagulation; NBM: nil by mouth

Source: Reprinted by permission from Macmillan Publishers Ltd: Journal of Perinatology. 23 (3), 200-204. Lima-Rogel, V., Calhoun, D. A., Maheshwari, A., Torres-Montes, A., Roque-Sanchez, R., Garcia, M. G., & Christensen, R. D. Tolerance of a Sterile Isotonic Electrolyte Solution Containing Select Recombinant Growth Factors in Neonates Recovering From Necrotizing Enterocolitis, copyright (2003).

Box 2.35   Acute gastrointestinal obstruction – CHECKLIST

Common/classic signs

- Bilious vomiting/aspirates
- Abdominal distension
- Failure to pass meconium/stool ('ileus')

Immediate interventions

- NBM
- Gastric decompression
- IV fluids

Then ...

- Referral to surgical team
- Pain control

(continued)

- Respiratory support
- Cardiovascular support
- Parent care, explanation and support

Subsequent care will depend on whether the neonate is managed medically or surgically. (de la Hunt, 2006)

See also *Surgical nursing practice*

Check local guidance for the assessment, care and referral procedures for the neonate with NEC or any other form of GIT obstruction

---

 Management should commence as early as possible once any suspicion of NEC or acute intestinal obstruction arises (Parker, 2013).

 Stop and think   **Standard precautions**

 Local variations   **Signposts**

 Always apply thorough infection control when handling or preparing any milk product, feeding or administering total parenteral nutrition (TPN) to a neonate.

The space below can be used to record any local variations and practice points specific to your own unit.

Gastrointestinal care: Glossary

Colostrum: The first secretion from the breasts after giving birth which is rich in antibodies and nutrients.

Expressed breast milk: Breast milk that has been extracted using a hand or breast pump. It contains both hind and foremilk and will be frozen to give to a neonate at a later time when they are able to take enteral feeds.

Formula milk: Manufactured modification of cow's milk designed and marketed for feeding to neonates.

Gastrostomy: Surgically created opening in the stomach through which a neonate can be fed if they cannot be fed via the usual oral route.

Gavage feeding: Feeding through a tube placed into the nose or mouth and passed down into the stomach.

Lactation: The secretion of breast milk by the breasts.

Total parenteral nutrition (TPN): The administration of a nutritionally complete solution given intravenously when it is not possible to feed enterally.

Trophic feeding: A small volume of balanced enteral nutrition insufficient for actual nutritional needs but producing some positive gastrointestinal benefit. Also called minimal enteral nutrition.

The Glossaries for *Fluid balance and electrolytes* and *Surgical nursing practices* are also relevant for this section.

Gastrointestinal care: References

Cirgin Ellett, M.L., Cohen, M.D., Perkins, S.M., Croffie, J., Lane, K.A., and Austin, J.K. (2012). Comparing methods of determining insertion length for placing gastric tubes in children 1 month to 17 years of age. *Journal for Specialists in Pediatric Nursing*. 17 (1): 19–32.

de la Hunt M.N. (2006). The acute abdomen in the newborn. *Seminars in Fetal and Neonatal Medicine*. 11 (3): 191–197.

East of England Perinatal Network (EEPN) (2012). *Nutrition Care Pathway*. East of England (EOE) Neonatal Operational Delivery Network (ODN): Cambridge

ElHassan, N.O. and Kaiser, J.R. (2011). Parenteral nutrition in the neonatal intensive care unit. *Neo Reviews*. 12: e130–140.

Embleton, N.D. (2013). Optimal nutrition for preterm infants: Putting the ESPGHAN guidelines into practice. *Journal of Neonatal Nursing*. 19 (4): 130–133.

Gephart, S.M., McGrath, J.M., Effken, J.A., Halpern, M.D. (2012). Necrotizing enterocolitis risk: State of the science. *Adv. Neonatal Care*. 12 (2):77–87.

Henderson, G., Anthony, M.Y., and McGuire, W. (2007). Formula milk versus maternal breast milk for feeding preterm or low birth weight infants. *Cochrane Database of Systematic Reviews*. Issue 4. Art. No.: CD002972.

Johnson, P.J. (2014). Review of macronutrients in parenteral nutrition for neonatal intensive care population. *Neonatal Network*. 33 (1): 29–40.

Kempley, S., Neelam, G., Linsell, L., Dorling, J., McCormick, K., Mannix, P., Juszczak, E., Brocklehurst, P., and Leaf, A. (2014). Feeding infants below 29 weeks' gestation with abnormal antenatal Doppler: Analysis from a randomised trial. *Arch Dis Child Fetal Neonatal Ed*. 99 (1): F6–F11.

King, C. (2005). Human milk for preterm infants – When and how to fortify. *Infant*. 1 (2): 44–46, 48.

Kuschel, C.A. and Harding, J.E. (2004). Multicomponent fortified human milk for promoting growth in preterm infants. *Cochrane Database of Systematic Reviews*. Issue 1. Art. No.: CD000343.

Laukaityte, A. (2013). Neonatal necrotising enterocolitis – Fact sheet. *Journal of Neonatal Nursing*. 19 (2): 54–57.

Leaf, A., Dorling, J., Kempley, S., McCormick, K., Mannix, P., Linsell, L., Juszczak, E., Brocklehurst, P., on behalf of the Abnormal Doppler Enteral Prescription Trial Collaborative Group. (2012). Early or Delayed Enteral Feeding for Preterm Growth-Restricted Infants: A randomized trial. *Pediatrics*. 129 (5), e1260–e1268.

Morgan, J., Bombell, S., and McGuire, W. (2013). Early trophic feeding versus enteral fasting for very preterm or very low birth weight infants. *Cochrane Database of Systematic Reviews*. Issue 3. Art. No.: CD000504.

NICE (2007). MCN consultation: Expert Report – Handling and storage of expressed breast milk. http://www.nice.org.uk/guidance/index.jsp?action=download&o=34694.

NHS. (2012). Guide to bottle feeding, London: NHS. Available at: www.nhs.uk/start4life

National Patient Safety Association (2005). Reducing the harm caused by misplaced naso- and orogastric feeding tubes in babies under the care of neonatal units. http://www.nrls.npsa.nhs.uk/EasySiteWeb/getresource.axd?AssetID=60018&

Nyqvist, K. H., Häggkvist, A. P., Hansen, M. N., Kylberg, E., Frandsen, A. L., Maastrup, R., & Haiek, L. N. (2013). Expansion of the Baby-Friendly Hospital Initiative Ten Steps to Successful Breastfeeding into Neonatal Intensive Care Expert Group Recommendations. *Journal of Human Lactation* (online)http://jhl.sagepub.com/content/early/2013/05/30/0890334413489775.full.pdf+html

Parker, L. (2013). Necrotizing enterocolitis: Have we made any progress in reducing the risk? *Advances in Neonatal Care*. 13 (5): 317–324.

Royal College of Nursing. (2013). Formula feeds: RCN guidance for nurses caring for infants and mothers. RCN: London. http://www.rcn.org.uk/__data/assets/pdf_file/0009/78741/003137.PDF

Schulzke, S.M., Deshpande, G.C., and Patole, S.K. (2007). Neurodevelopmental outcomes of very low-birth-weight infants with necrotizing enterocolitis: A systematic review of observational studies. *Arch Pediatr Adolesc Med*. 161: 583–590.

Tho, P. C., Mordiffi, S., Ang, E. and Chen, H. (2011), Implementation of the evidence review on best practice for confirming the correct placement of nasogastric tube in patients in an acute care hospital. *International Journal of Evidence-Based Healthcare*, 9: 51–60.

UK Department of Health and Food Standards Agency (2011). Guidelines on preparation of powdered milk formula. http://www.food.gov.uk/multimedia/pdfs/formulaguidance.pdf

UNICEF (2013). Off to the best start. http://www.unicef.org.uk/BabyFriendly/Resources/Resources-for-parents/Off-to-the-best-start/

WHO (in collaboration with FAO) (2007). Guidelines for the safe preparation, storage and handling of powdered infant formula. www.who.int/foodsafety/publications/micro/pif2007/en/index.html

Further reading: neonatal nutrition

A sound body of theory underpins this topic and the reader may refer to the following selected open access resources to explore this further.

Giannì, M.L., Roggero, P., Colnaghi, M.R., Piemontese, P., Amato, O., Orsi, A., and Mosca, F. (2014). The role of nutrition in promoting growth in pre-term infants with bronchopulmonary dysplasia: A prospective non-randomised interventional cohort study. *BMC Paediatrics*. 14 (1): 235. http://www.biomedcentral.com/1471-2431/14/235.

Puntis, J. (2006). Nutritional support in the premature newborn. *Postgraduate Medicine Journal*. 82 (965): 192–198. http://www.ncbi.nlm.nih.gov/pmc/articles/PMC2563699/

Clark, R.H., Wagner, C.L., Merritt, R.J., Bloom, B.T., Neu, J., Young, T.E., and Clark, D.A. (2003). Nutrition in the neonatal intensive care unit: How do we reduce the incidence of extrauterine growth restriction? *Journal of Perinatology*. 23 (4): 337–344. http://www.nature.com/jp/journal/v23/n4/full/7210937a.html

The three Hs (metabolic triangle) and hygiene needs

This chapter representing 'H' covers two different topics; one is termed the 'three Hs' (hypoxia, hypothermia and hypoglycaemia) or what is known as the 'metabolic triangle' (Aylott, 2006a, 2006b) and the second is hygiene needs in the neonate.

The three Hs – (the metabolic triangle)

At birth, the neonate undergoes the transition from the *in utero* to the *ex utero* environment and must adapt from being a fetus to a neonate who lives independently from the mother and from the placental transfusion of oxygen and nutrition (Askin, 2009). Successful transition depends on the availability of adequate oxygen, energy in the form of glucose and satisfactory thermal control (Platt and Deshpande, 2005). This occurs in the majority of neonates when born healthy. However, when compromise ensues in the perinatal period, one, two or all of these three elements may be deficient, leading to the potential for hypoxia, hypoglycaemia and/or hypothermia (Knoebel, 2014). Moreover, each element influences the other. This is depicted in Figures 2.22a and 2.22b .

> Related topics: See also *Airway* and *Assessment*, *Breathing* and *Oxygen therapy* for sections relevant to hypoxia. In addition, see *Blood/blood taking* for information on blood glucose analysis and hypoglycaemia and *Thermal care* for information relating to the prevention of hypothermia.

Figure 2.22a The metabolic triangle: the well neonate at birth – DIAGRAM

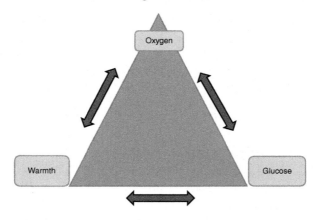

Source: Printed from Aylott, M (2006), The neonatal energy triangle part 1: Metabolic adaptation. Paediatric Nursing. 18 (6). Pages 38-42, with permission from Nursing Children and Young People journal (formerly Paediatric Nursing).

The neonate requires early provision of all three of these areas for successful adaptation to extrauterine life, from delivery room and thereafter.

Figure 2.22b The relationship between the three Hs: compromise at birth – DIAGRAM

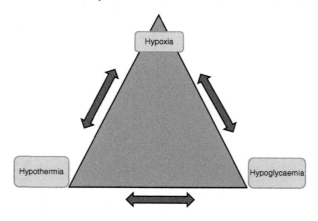

The best rule of thumb is prevention of any part of the triangle by simple, basic care measures (e.g. early nutrition, avoidance of heat loss and maintaining adequate oxygenation).

The relationship explained....

Hypothermia causes an increase in glucose use, which can lead to hypoglycaemia and increased utilization of oxygen to heat the body, which can lead to hypoxia (Fawcett, 2014)

Hypoxia depletes oxygen for basic functions such as glucose metabolism and thermogenesis, which can lead to hypoglycaemia and hypothermia

Hypoglycaemia depletes glucose for basic functions such as respiratory function and thermal control which can lead to hypoxia and hypothermia

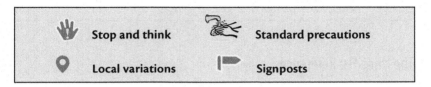

Ensure standard precautions are upheld in the early care of any neonate in conjunction with these important areas of practice to minimise infection risk.

The space below can be used to record any local variations and practice points specific to your own unit.

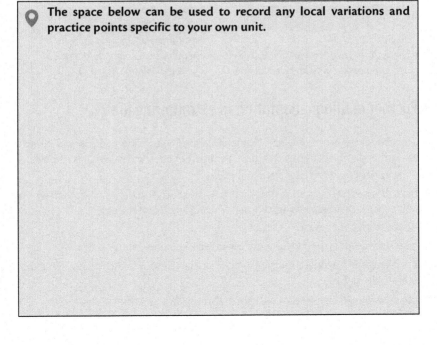

The three Hs: Glossary

Fetus: Period from start of week nine in pregnancy until birth.

Metabolic adaptation: The transition that occurs after birth as the newborn changes from being within the *in utero* environment to the extrauterine environment.

Neonate: Period of life up to 28 days post-term.

Perinatal period: The time immediately before and after birth.

> The Glossaries for *Airway, Assessment, Breathing, Blood/blood taking, Oxygen Therapy and Thermal care* are also relevant for this topic.

The three Hs: References

*Askin, D.F. (2009). Fetal to neonatal transition – What is normal and what is not? *Neonatal Network*. 28 (3): e33–e40.

*Aylott, M. (2006a). The neonatal energy triangle part 1; Metabolic adaptation. *Paediatric Nursing*. 18 (6): 38–42.

*Aylott, M. (2006b). The neonatal energy triangle part 2; Thermoregulatory and respiratory adaptation. *Paediatric Nursing*. 18 (7): 38–43.

Fawcett, K. (2014). Preventing admission hypothermia in very low birthweight neonates. *Neonatal Network*. 33 (3): 143–149.

*Knobel, R.B. (2014). Thermal stability of the premature infant in neonatal intensive care. *Newborn and Infant Nursing Reviews*. 14 (2):72–76. http://www.medscape.com/viewarticle/826082.

*Platt, M.W. and Deshpande, S. (2005). Metabolic adaptation at birth. *Seminars in Fetal and Neonatal Medicine*. 10 (4): 341–350.

Further reading: adaptation to extrauterine life

The above documents marked * contain detailed information and should be read for further depth relating to this topic. Some other open access web links are below.

University of Hertfordshire Neonatal page

http://www.herts.ac.uk/apply/schools-of-study/health-and-social-work/course-subject-areas/nursing/childrens-nursing/neonatal-nursing.

Anaesthesia UK Foetal Circulation

http://www.frca.co.uk/Documents/Foetal%20circulation.pdf

Knowledge for neonatal nursing practice online resource: Adaptation to extrauterine life

http://www.cetl.org.uk/learning/neonatal/unit_2c/player.html.

Hygiene needs and care

Even the sickest neonate requires their basic hygiene needs attended to. This area is a prime example of the care practices that can be offered and taught to parents in the neonatal unit (NNU) to encourage participation in care. Figure 2.23 and Box 2.36 outline the main care principles for a range of hygiene practices.

Related topics: see also *Skin care. Umbilical care and catheters* is also relevant for this specific area.

During care procedures is an ideal time to assess skin integrity (Allwood, 2011).

Figure 2.23   Principles of hygiene care in the neonate – FLOW CHART

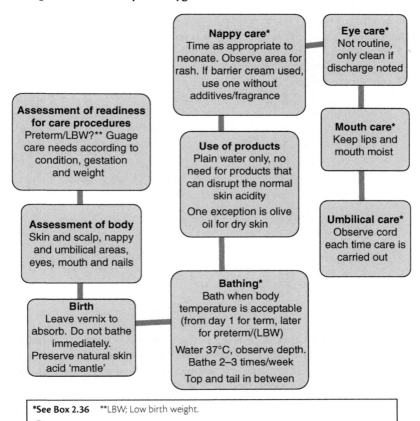

Nappy care*
Time as appropriate to neonate. Observe area for rash. If barrier cream used, use one without additives/fragrance

Eye care*
Not routine, only clean if discharge noted

Assessment of readiness for care procedures
Preterm/LBW?** Guage care needs according to condition, gestation and weight

Mouth care*
Keep lips and mouth moist

Use of products
Plain water only, no need for products that can disrupt the normal skin acidity
One exception is olive oil for dry skin

Assessment of body
Skin and scalp, nappy and umbilical areas, eyes, mouth and nails

Umbilical care*
Observe cord each time care is carried out

Birth
Leave vernix to absorb. Do not bathe immediately. Preserve natural skin acid 'mantle'

Bathing*
Bath when body temperature is acceptable (from day 1 for term, later for preterm/(LBW)
Water 37°C, observe depth. Bathe 2–3 times/week
Top and tail in between

*See Box 2.36   ******LBW; Low birth weight.

Check local guidance for care practices relating to hygiene

> ***Box 2.36   Hygiene needs in the neonate: additional practice points –**
> CHECKLIST
>
> - Gather all items required including gloves and disposal bag.
> - **Nappy care:** Change nappy at intervals according to the neonate's
>   condition and need. Use water only and possibly use a thin layer of barrier
>   cream. Observe nappy area closely. If a rash is present, expose if possible and
>   topical treatment may be required.
> - **Bathing:** Time according to gestation, weight and ability to maintain
>   temperature. Bath water temperature should be 37°C; depth no more than
>   2–3 cm. There is no need to use any products. Wash hair first keeping
>   neonate wrapped and then expose body to place in bath. Observe tolerance
>   and watch for signs of stress. Lift neonate safely by placing your arm under
>   their body, clasping their far upper arm firmly and holding both ankles with
>   your other hand.
> - **Top and tail:** Face and nappy area only.
> - **Eye care:** Not routine, perform only if discharge noted. Use sterile gauze,
>   one piece for each eye and use sterile water; sweep inwards to outwards,
>   discarding each piece of gauze after each sweep.
> - **Mouth care:** Use soft sponges or cotton buds to clean mouth with water
>   and keep lips and tongue moist.
> - **Umbilical cord care:** Once cut and clamped (after 1 minute in well
>   neonates; or immediately in unwell/unstable neonates) keep stump exposed
>   above nappy, keep dry except when bathing. Only use water to clean the
>   area around stump. Ensure the stump dries up and separates by 10–14 days.
>   If any redness or discharge, send swab and refer for possible antibiotics.
>
> Standard precautions should be applied to any hygiene practice
> involving bodily fluids to prevent cross infection to neonates, families and staff.
>
> Check local guidance for hygiene practices
>
> *References:* Zupan et al. (2004); Mainstone (2005); Blincoe (2006); Jackson (2008);
> Trotter (2008, 2013); Atherton (2009); Visscher (2009); Petty (2012); Elser (2013);
> NICE (2013).

> **Parents may choose to bring in their own products such as baby
> wipes, soaps or olive oil. They should be advised that products must
> have a neutral pH. In the hospital setting, generally water is used alone
> with products being prescribed only if necessary, for example, in the
> case of nappy rash or skin excoriation. ▶ See *Skin care.***

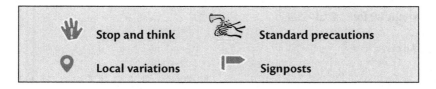

Stop and think   Standard precautions

Local variations   Signposts

Always wear gloves when handling any body fluids during care procedures and wash hands thoroughly before and afterwards.

The space below can be used to record any local variations and practice points specific to your own unit.

Hygiene needs: Glossary

All cares: Referring to the full repertoire of care practices necessary for personal hygiene including nappy care, mouth care, top and tail/bathing, umbilical care.

Barrier cream: A topical agent used as a barrier on the nappy area to prevent irritation from urine and stool.

Changing stool: The normal seedy stool that is first seen after the neonate has passed meconium and is established on feeding.

Emollient: A substance that softens and moisturizes the skin.

Meconium: Fetal stool. The thick, sticky and dark green substance forming the first faeces of a newborn baby.

> The Glossaries for *Skin care* and *Umbilical care and catheters* are also relevant for this topic.

Hygiene needs: References

Allwood, M. (2011). Skincare guidelines for infants aged 23–30 weeks gestation: A review of the literature. *Neonatal, Paediatric and Child Health Nursing.* 14 (1): 20.

Atherton, D.J. (2009). Managing healthy skin for babies. *Infant.* 5 (4): 130–132.

Blincoe, A.J. (2006). Caring for neonatal skin and common infant skin problems. *British Journal of Midwifery.* 14 (4): 213–216

Elser, H. (2013). Bathing basics: How clean should neonates be? *Advances in Neonatal Care.* 13 (3): 188–189.

Jackson, A. (2008). Time to review newborn skin care. *Infant.* 4 (5): 168–171.

Mainstone, A. (2005). Maintaining infant skin health and hygiene. *British Journal of Midwifery.* 13 (1): 44–47.

NICE Clinical Knowledge Summary. (2013). Nappy Rash. http://www.cks.nhs.uk/nappy_rash

Petty, J.D. (2012). Personal hygiene and pressure ulcer prevention. In S. Macqueen, E. Bruce, and F. Gibson, (Eds), *The Great Ormond Street Hospital Manual of Children's Nursing Practices.* Oxford, Wiley-Blackwell.

Trotter, S. (2008). Neonatal skin and cord care – The way forward. *Nursing in Practice.* 40: 40–45.

Trotter, S. (2013). Why no baby skincare product should be advertised or promoted as 'suitable for new-born skin'. *MIDIRS Midwifery Digest.* 23 (2): 217–221.

Visscher, M. (2009). Update on the use of topical agents in neonates. *Newborn Infant Nurs Rev.* 9 (1): 31–47.

Zupan, J., Garner, P., and Omari, A.A.A. (2004). Topical umbilical cord care at birth. *Cochrane Database of Systematic Reviews.* Issue 3. Art. No.: CD001057. DOI: 10.1002/14651858.CD001057.pub2.

Infection and immunizations

This chapter covers the very important issue of infection in neonatal care including immunizations.

Immaturity and illness make neonates vulnerable to infection and it is imperative that measures are taken to prevent it. Standard precautions must be adhered to at all times, which includes hand hygiene, protective clothing, sharps and waste disposal, management of equipment and environment and the safe care of linen including uniforms (UK Dept. of Health, 2009; RCN, 2012; UK Government, 2012).

> The theme of standard precautions and prevention of infection has been threaded throughout this book with regular reminders and is therefore relevant to *all* chapters.

It is worth reiterating that thorough hand washing is vital. The World Health Organization's (WHO, 2006) Five Moments for hand hygiene should be followed, as outlined below.

Five moments for hand hygiene

Before touching a patient
Before clean and aseptic procedures
After contact with body fluids
After touching a patient
After touching patient surroundings

Figure 2.24 covers an overview of neonatal sepsis and what makes up the neonatal septic screen. Table 2.22 provides a synopsis of the UK recommended immunization programme.

Understanding neonatal sepsis and the septic screen

Early diagnosis and treatment of the neonate with suspected infection are essential to prevent long-term complications associated with systemic sepsis (Short, 2004) and to treat appropriately with antibiotics, if necessary, in a timely fashion (Johnston and Anthony, 2013). It is essential to have an understanding of the risk factors and clinical signs, as well as the haematological markers. Diagnosis and the decision to start antibiotics is based on a combination of factors and is undertaken on an individual basis.

Figure 2.24 Identifying neonatal infection and the septic screen – DIAGRAM

Early onset
- **Early onset infection (within 72 hours).**
- **Identify risk factors:**
- **Maternal signs:** Fever, high C reactive protien (CRP), offensive amniotic fluid, antibiotics required before/during labour.
- **Neonatal 'Red flag' signs:** At risk for Group B streptococcus, prolonged rupture of membranes, preterm birth, fever > 38 degrees Celcius, respiratory distress, need for ventilation, shock.

Late onset
- **Late onset infection (after 72 hours).**
- **Identify risk factors:**
- Central venous catheterisation, invasive procedures, lines, tubes and IV sites, ventilation or CPAP, humidification, steroid therapy, poor nutrition, poor skin integrity, poor hand hygiene and hand washing practices

Septic screen
- **Septic screen: Can be taken in full or partial; i.e. all or some of the following tests may be undertaken (NICE, 2012)**
- **Haematological:** Blood culture before antibiotics, CRP, full blood count particularly white cell count and neutrophils, platelets, urea and electrolytes, clotting times, lactate, glucose.
- **Swabs as appropriate:** For example, umbilicus, skin, ear.
- **X- ray:** Chest, abdominal
- **Urine sample:** Bag or suprapubic
- **Lumbar puncture:** If there is a strong indication of neurological risk or involvement

Strict infection control by adhering to Standard precautions as described previously and in the Glossary is an integral component of this area of care. This is essential to prevent any further risk of infection to the neonate.

Check local guidance for septic screen policy and specific practices

References: Short (2004); Arnon and Litmanovitx (2008); Hawk (2008); NICE, (2012); Berardi et al. (2013); Johnston and Anthony (2013); Ismail and Gandhi (2014)

In any neonate that deteriorates, infection should always be considered as a potential diagnosis and a septic screen commenced as soon as possible (Abdelrhim et al., 2014).

Immunizations

This unit outlines the latest Childhood Immunization Schedule from the NHS.

For full schedule including all age groups and risk groups see Public Health England (2014: https://www.gov.uk/government/collections/immunisation).

Table 2.22   Immunization Schedule (up to school age) – SUMMARY TABLE

Age due	Immunization (s)	Route
8 weeks	DTaP/IPV/Hib PCV	IM thigh
12 weeks	DTaP/IPV/Hib Men C Rotavirus	IM thigh Mouth
16 weeks	DTaP/IPV/Hib PCV	IM thigh
12–13 months	Hib Men C PCV MMR (1st)	IM thigh or arm
2 and 3 years	Influenza	Nasal spray or arm
3 years 4 months (pre-school)	MMR (2nd) DTaP/IPV or dTaP/IPV	IM arm IM arm
Immunizations for at - risk groups		
Birth, 1, 2 and 12 months	Hep B	IM thigh
Birth	TB	Upper arm (intradermal)
6 months up to 2 years	Inactivated Influenza (prior to influenza season)	IM thigh or arm

Key:
DTaP   Diphtheria, Tetanus, acellular Pertussis
IPV   Inactivated Polio Vaccine
Hib   Haemophilus influenzae b
PCV   Pneumococcal
Men C   Meningococcal C
MMR   Measles, Mumps, Rubella
dT   low dose Diptheria, tetanus
dTaP   low dose Diphtheria, Tetanus, acellular Pertussis
Hep B   Hepatitis B
TB   Tuberculosis

Reference: Public Health England (2014)

Neonates born prematurely should be immunized in line with the recommended schedule from two months after birth, no matter how premature they were born. However, if they are in the neonatal unit, they should be free from any infection and their condition deemed fit enough to undertake immunization.

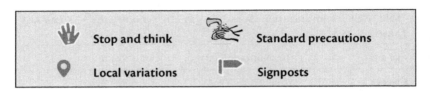

Stop and think   Standard precautions

Local variations   Signposts

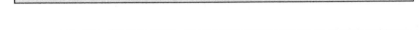

Infection prevention is a key theme running through this whole book.

The space below can be used to record any local variations and practice points specific to your own unit.

Infection control and immunizations: Glossary

Aseptic non-touch technique (ANTT): A method by which precautions are taken during clinical procedures to prevent the transfer of microorganisms to the patient by the avoidance of touching key parts that come into direct contact with them.

C-reactive protein (CRP): A protein that is a by-product of acute inflammation.

Culture: A microbiological analysis of blood to identify infections, specific pathogens and resistance to antibiotic agents.

Lumbar puncture: A procedure whereby a needle is used to extract cerebrospinal fluid (CSF) from the subarachnoid space within the spinal cord to assess the presence of infection.

Infection: (or sepsis: see below) General term for invasion from a pathogen, either bacterial, viral or fungal. Some examples are:

Group B streptococcus: A bacterial infection that a neonate can contract as he/she passes through an infected birth canal, sometimes resulting in severe illness.

Chickenpox (varicella): A common childhood viral illness characterized by itchy spots and fever. When contracted by a pregnant woman, it can occasionally cause birth defects or severe newborn illness.

Coagulase-negative Staphylococcus (CONS): A frequent blood culture isolate in the neonate. This can be a blood culture contaminant but can also be a significant cause of infection.

Cytomegalovirus: A viral infection that, when contracted by a pregnant woman, can result in severe newborn illness, and sometimes lead to chronic disabilities such as learning difficulties, vision and hearing loss.

Escherichia coli: A Gram-negative bacteria that is commonly found in the lower intestine.

Herpes simplex: A virus that can be transmitted sexually, sometimes causing genital sores in infected adults. A neonate may become infected passing through an infected birth canal, sometimes resulting in severe newborn illness or future medical problems.

Human immunodeficiency virus (HIV): A retrovirus that destroys helper T cells of the immune system causing the marked reduction in their numbers and significant immune compromise.

Listeria: A type of bacteria which infects humans through contaminated food.

Staphylococcus: A bacteria that includes many pathogenic kinds that cause pus formation, especially in the skin and mucous membranes. A common cause of neonatal postnatal infection. See CONS above and MRSA below.

Methicillin resistant Staphylococcus aureus (MRSA): A strain of Staphylococcus that has become resistant to antibiotics.

Respiratory syncytial virus (RSV): A virus which causes infection of the respiratory tract. It is a major cause of bronchiolitis and pneumonia in young children.

Toxoplasmosis: A parasitic infection that, when contracted by a pregnant woman, can result in serious newborn illness and chronic disabilities.

Meningitis: Inflammation / infection of the meninges (linings) of the brain and spinal cord.

Sepsis: Any evidence of infection requiring antibiotic therapy, which is confirmed with a blood culture. Septicaemia is where there is a potentially dangerous invasion of a pathogen into the bloodstream, which indicates that an infection has become systemic.

Septic screen: A set of tests carried out when infection is suspected: includes blood culture, blood C-reactive protein (CRP), full blood count and electrolytes, swabs and urine testing for microbiology. Sometimes a lumbar puncture is carried out.

Standard precautions: A set of basic infection prevention practices intended to prevent transmission of infectious diseases from one person to another. These precautions were formerly known as 'universal precautions.'

TORCH infection: The mneumonic that describes a range of pathogens that can cause congenital infection. The letters represent: 'Toxoplasmosis', 'Other' (Chicken pox (Varicella), HIV, Parainfluenza), 'Rubella', 'Cytomegalovirus', 'Herpes'.

Infection control and immunizations: References

Abdelrhim, H., Heaton, P.A., Routley, C., and Paul, S.P. (2014). Treatment for early-onset neonatal sepsis. *Nursing Times.* 110 (14): 24–25.

Arnon, S. and Litmanovitz, I. (2008). Diagnostic tests in neonatal sepsis. *Current Opinion in Infectious Diseases.* 21(3): 223–227.

Berardi, A., Rossi, C., Lugli, L., Creti, R., Reggiani, M.L.B., Lanari, M., and Ferrari, F. (2013). Group B streptococcus late-onset disease: 2003–2010. *Pediatrics.* 131 (2): e361–e368.

Hawk, M. (2008). C-reactive protein in neonatal sepsis. *Neonatal Network.* 27 (2): 117–120.

Ismail, A.Q. and Gandhi, A. (2014). Using CRP in neonatal practice. *Journal of Maternal-Fetal Neonatal Medicine.* 28 (1): 3–6.

Johnston, S.E. and Anthony, M. (2013). Antibiotics for early onset neonatal infection. *Archives of Disease in Childhood: Fetal Neonatal Edition.* 98 (2): F184–185.

NICE. (2012). *Antibiotics for early-onset neonatal infection* (CG149). http://guidance.nice.org.uk/CG149.

Public Health England (2014). *Immunisation Schedule.* https://www.gov.uk/government/collections/immunisation.

RCN (2012). *Essential practice for infection prevention and control; Guidance for nursing staff.* London: RCN.

Short, M.A. (2004). Guide to a systematic physical assessment in the infant with suspected infection and/or sepsis. *Advances in Neonatal Care.* 4 (3):141–153.

UK Department of Health (2009). *The Health and Social Care Act 2008: Code of practice for health and adult social care on the prevention and control of infections and related guidance.* London: DH.

UK Government (2012). *Save lives: Clean your hands.* https://www.gov.uk/government/news/save-lives-clean-your-hands.

WHO. (2006). *WHO Guidelines on Hand Hygiene in Health Care.* http://whqlibdoc.who.int/publications/2009/9789241597906_eng.pdf. http://www.who.int/gpsc/tools/Five_moments/en/.

Jaundice

This chapter focuses on a common neonatal condition, jaundice, the well-known term for hyperbilirubinaemia (Truman, 2006; Turnbull and Petty, 2012).

It is cited that up to two thirds of all neonates will exhibit clinical signs of jaundice in the first few weeks of life (Rennie et al., 2010; Schwartz et al., 2011) and this number increases in the preterm neonate due to immaturity of bilirubin metabolism. The units covered in this chapter (Tables 2.23a–b–2.25, Figure 2.25, and Boxes 2.37–2.38a–b) cover measurement of bilirubin, assessing different types of jaundice, methods and care of phototherapy and an overview of exchange blood transfusion required when phototherapy is no longer effective as a treatment option.

Related topics: see also *Assessment* to view how jaundice is assessed in the context of all the systems and *Blood/blood taking* for information on other important blood tests that are commonplace in neonatal care.

Measuring and assessing bilirubin levels

Serum bilirubin measurement (SBR) is not recommended routinely for those neonates without visible jaundice. However, within the neonatal unit, neonates are more likely to be jaundiced and so bilirubin measurement is commonly done. This unit summarizes the assessment of jaundice and bilirubin measurement

Table 2.23a   Methods of assessing for the presence of jaundice –
SUMMARY TABLE

Clinical observation	Transcutaneous (TcB) (skin)	Serum bilirubin (SBR)
View the neonate naked in good, natural light. Observe the sclera, oral mucosa and blanched skin for the presence of yellow discolouration (Ford, 2010) Continue to observe regularly during times when the neonate is being attended to for their basic care needs. Parents may also note their neonate appears jaundiced. This method should not be relied on solely particularly in any neonate who is slow to feed or has any other risk factors such as prematurity or infection.	The sternum or the forehead can be used for application of a non-invasive transcutaneous probe for near-term babies *after* the first 24 hours and for neonates born >35 weeks gestation only This method offers a non-invasive way of assessing bilirubin that is hand-held and portable. Readings above 250 micromol/l are unreliable however and so SBR should be used in this situation (NICE, 2010, 2012) (Sarici et al., 2014) The company guidelines for this device should be followed.	A serum bilirubin is measured, taken by capillary, venous or arterial routes. A sample taken in a heparinized capillary tube can be processed at ward level using a bilirubinometer for analysis of *total* bilirubin. To assess the *split* between conjugated and unconjugated bilirubin, blood is sent to the laboratory. The SBR method is used when TcB method is not available or appropriate, for neonates less than 24 hours old where visible jaundice is present and for any neonate born at less than 35 weeks gestation. For jaundice in the first 24 hours, SBR should be taken within 2 hours. Use SBR method for any neonate where bilirubin is above treatment threshold.

Observe local guidance for agreed methods of bilirubin monitoring.

Visible inspection alone should not be used to estimate a neonate's bilirubin level.

Table 2.23b   Bilirubin thresholds and actions (Term >38 weeks gestation) – SUMMARY TABLE

Age (hours)	Bilirubin (micromol/l)			
0 ⇩	>100	>112	>100	>100
96	>200	>300	>350	>450
Plot all measurements on correct treatment threshold graph according to gestation				
ACTIONS	Repeat bilirubin measurement in 6–12 hours	Consider phototherapy. Repeat bilirubin in 6 hours	Start phototherapy. Single first and then consider double/triple if bilirubin remains high	Consider exchange transfusion after double or triple phototherapy has been given

📍 Along with national guidance from NICE (see below), check local guidance on specific aspects of assessment and care of the jaundiced neonate

References: NICE (2010, 2012)

🖐 **Refer to the NICE full guidance on neonatal jaundice for all treatment threshold graphs for all gestational ages. Preterm neonates have a lowered threshold for starting treatment (Ford, 2010; Turnbull and Petty, 2012; O'Conner et al., 2013).**

Assessing types of jaundice

The Glossary for this section defines the three types of jaundice: physiological, pathological and prolonged. For physiological and pathological jaundice, the cause is usually known and bilirubin is an unconjugated form treated with phototherapy. However, for prolonged jaundice, it is important to distinguish if it is due to unconjugated or conjugated bilirubin (Tyler and McKiernan, 2006). In addition, cause needs to be ascertained, as this may be indicative of a potential and serious disease condition (e.g. cholestasis). This unit covers the types of jaundice including what a prolonged jaundice screen involves.

Table 2.24 Types of neonatal jaundice – SUMMARY TABLE		
Jaundice type (see Glossary)	**Onset/timing**	**Type of bilirubin**
Physiological	After day 3 to day 7 approximately	Unconjugated
Pathological	Within the first 24 hours	Unconjugated
Prolonged	Persists past the usual 7–10 day period	Conjugated or unconjugated

> ✋ **Breast-milk jaundice should be a consideration in the presence of prolonged jaundice which is not due to a disease process.**

Box 2.37   Prolonged jaundice screen – CHECKLIST

Blood tests
- Total and conjugated serum bilirubin- A 'split bili' blood test differentiates between the two types of bilirubin
- Full blood count, blood group, direct antibody test and urine culture
- Liver function tests
- Thyroxine and thyroid-stimulating hormone
- Galactosaemia screen

Urine
- Microscopy, culture and sensitivity
- Reducing sugars (e.g. loss of galactose)
- Look for dark urine that stains the nappy

Stool
- Stool specimen in an opaque pot – look for pale chalky stools

Other
- Ensure that routine metabolic screening has been performed
- Infection screen including congenital infection and hepatitis

Follow expert advice about care for neonates with a conjugated bilirubin level greater than 25 micromol/l.

 Observe local guidance on prolonged jaundice screening.

> ✋ **Prolonged jaundice may be indicative of a serious disease that requires treatment. Therefore, assessment and monitoring are vital.**

Phototherapy

The main treatment for significant jaundice is phototherapy, which converts unconjugated bilirubin to a conjugated, safe form that can be excreted. This unit summarizes the different types in clinical use.

Table 2.25 Phototherapy devices – SUMMARY TABLE	
Conventional	**Fibre optic**
Light source delivered via halogen bulb, fluorescent lamps or light emitting diodes. Distance of light varies depending on model: range 25–50 cm from neonate	Light is passed through a fibre optic bundle and is placed next to the skin e.g. biliblanket or bed/mattress
Combination	
• Use both conventional and fibre optic together to increase irradiance of light • Double or triple phototherapy can be used to increase effectiveness (using two or three different devices to increase light sources)	
Requirements for effective phototherapy	
• An effective spectrum of light – in blue range (intensity 400–520 nm) • Sufficient irradiance of light – a measure of the amount of light reaching the skin • Maximum exposure of skin surface area to the phototherapy light • Metalloporphyrins may be used as a preventative measure	

Double or triple phototherapy should be attempted where high levels of SBR are present to avoid an exchange transfusion being administered (Box 2.38a).

Figure 2.25 Care of the neonate receiving phototherapy – DIAGRAM

SKIN
Expose as much skin as possible to increase irradiance of light
No creams on skin or nappy area

PARENTS
Explain to, and support parents. Consider time off lights if appropriate

EYES
Cover eyes to protect retina

Phototherapy

FLUIDS
If possible, feed as normal. Assess fluid status* and adjust requirements if applicable

COMFORT LEVELS
Assess for signs of stress and provide comfort measures

MONITORING
Monitor temperature** and other vital signs as applicable

Note: *Fluid balance: fluid requirements may need adjusting but not routinely

**Temperature: older phototherapy lights using bulb light sources emit heat while newer models may not. Conversely the neonate is exposed so may lose heat.

Aim: to provide a balance between normalizing care and reducing bilirubin levels as soon as possible.

 Observe local guidance on specific care practices

References: Mills and Tudehope (2001); Suresh et al. (2003); Kumar et al. (2011)

There is no evidence to prove that one form of phototherapy is more effective than another (Wentworth, 2005). Whatever device is used, the neonate must be cared for and monitored in the same way.

Exchange transfusion

When phototherapy is ineffective and bilirubin levels remain above the treatment threshold or continue to rise, a double volume exchange transfusion (DVET) will be necessary (NICE, 2010) where a proportion of the neonate's blood is exchanged with donor blood. Box 2.38a outlines a summary of this invasive procedure. 'Dilutional exchange' transfusion is also covered in Box 2.38b: this is when a proportion of blood is replaced with fluid in order to 'dilute' it, in the case of a high packed cell volume (PVC) known as polycythaemia.

Box 2.38a   Double volume exchange transfusion (DVET); Nursing care guide – FLOW CHART

DVET is used for treatment of severe hyperbilirubinaemia above the 'exchange line' on relevant charts, where bilirubin levels continue to rise steeply despite double and triple phototherapy (Thayyil and Milligan, 2006; NICE, 2010; 2012). The aim of DVET is to reduce the unconjugated bilirubin to a **safe level**, using twice the neonate's estimated blood volume (of 80mls/kg)

Obtain parental consent, preferably written.

Preparation and equipment

Insertion of lines: umbilical arterial and venous catheters (or occasionally peripheral in exceptional circumstances)

Equipment: blood warmer, blood (prescribed red cells for exchange blood transfusion, leucocyte depleted, CMV negative), warmed to 34–35°C, 10–20 ml syringes, three-way taps × 2, sterile pack, waste bag, sterile gown/gloves, IV tubing × 2

Checks: blood checked by two trained staff as per local policy. Line positions should be checked prior to starting the procedure.

Investigations: includes blood full blood count, urea and electrolytes, liver function, serum bilirubin, glucose, blood gas, clotting.

The procedure

Nurse in an open incubator in intensive care. Ensure NBM with an NGT inserted and kept on open drainage. Maintenance fluids should be commenced.

Two-catheter method: donor blood infused slowly through an umbilical venous catheter whilst the neonate's blood is removed via an umbilical artery catheter in timed aliquots of 5 ml/kg over 5 minutes.

Alternative method ('push-pull' using one large umbilical free-flowing catheter): 5 ml/kg of blood is aspirated slowly over 5 minutes, and then discarded. The same amount of blood from donor bag is pushed slowly into neonate. This completes a 5 minute cycle.

(continued)

▽
Monitoring and documentation

- Accurate fluid *balance* (input and output) should be maintained after each 5 ml cycle, ensuring that removed blood and transfused blood tally at all times. This balance should be checked at intervals throughout the whole procedure
- Document exact time exchange commenced and volumes infused and removed
- Continuously monitor and record pulse oximetry, heart rate, respiratory rate and blood pressure (invasive or cuff).
- Record baseline temperature and continue to check regularly
- Note any changes from the baseline
- Record all observations on the DVET chart with exact times
- Line checks – assess, dress and secure carefully

Post-transfusion management

- Check blood values again as stated previously, continue to monitor vital signs hourly, monitor serum bilirubin within two hours and regularly thereafter, keep lines in situ with heparin running through the arterial line.
- Continue phototherapy

 Remember standard precautions and strict asepsis at all times as this procedure is very invasive.

Observe local guidance for exchange transfusion procedures.

Source: Adapted with kind permission from Bart's Health Neonatal Unit, Royal London NHS Trust, London

References: NICE (2010; 2012); British Committee for Standards in Haematology (2004).

DVET is a very invasive procedure with potential complications such as circulatory overload or hypovolaemia, hypothermia due to unwarmed blood, cardiac arrhythmias (from hyperkalaemia), electrolyte disturbances, air embolism, catheter problems or NEC. In the event of a sudden collapse, stop the transfusion. A doctor or an advanced neonatal nurse practitioner carries out the exchange with a nurse providing one-to-one care.

Box 2.38b   Understanding dilutional exchange transfusion – FLOW CHART

The aim of the dilutional exchange is to reduce the packed cell volume (PCV) to 50–55% in the case of symptomatic polycythaemia. The neonate should be admitted to high dependency unit (HDU) or intensive care unit (ITU) and full vital signs monitoring commenced.

Ensure all relevant blood tests have been done including blood glucose, PCV and serum bilirubin.

Obtain venous and arterial access. An umbilical catheter is the easiest option for both.

Alternatively, a peripheral cannula inserted in a large vein and a peripheral arterial line can be used.

Normal saline is the replacement fluid of choice because it is inexpensive and effective.

The volume of blood to be diluted is calculated according to a formula. An example of one that could be used is below:

$$\text{Estimated blood volume} \quad \times \quad \frac{\text{Observed PCV} - \text{Desired PCV}}{\text{Observed PCV}}$$

The exchange should be done aseptically and aliquots of 5 ml/kg delivered and replaced over 5 minutes. Blood is removed through the arterial line and saline replaced via the venous line. If only a UVC is in place, the 'push-pull' technique can be used (See Box 2.38a).

Post-exchange, monitor vital signs for at least 24 hours and keep NBM. Check blood glucose, PCV, serum bilirubin, clotting screen and electrolyte levels.

 Observe local guidance for dilutional exchange criteria and procedure.

🖐 **Exchange transfusions are associated with risk and are invasive procedures. Therefore, *informed*, written consent should be obtained from parents.**

Stop and think   **Standard precautions**

 Local variations   **Signposts**

 Always apply principles when caring for any neonate with jaundice including wearing gloves when taking blood and ensuring that any equipment used for phototherapy is clean and dry. It is also absolutely essential to adhere to strict aseptic procedures for venous/arterial access and blood administration in relation to exchange transfusions.

 The space below can be used to record any local variations and practice points specific to your own unit.

Jaundice: Glossary

Bili-lights: The blue fluorescent phototherapy lights placed over a neonate's incubator used to treat jaundice.

Cholestasis: Stasis of the biliary system.

Exchange transfusion: A type of blood transfusion in which some of the neonate's blood is removed in small aliquots and replaced with donor blood; sometimes used to treat severe jaundice. May be used for hyperbilirubinaemia, haemolytic disease of the newborn and removal of toxins/drugs as in sepsis.

Hyperbilirubinaemia: High levels of circulating bilirubin in the blood. Bilirubin is produced from the breakdown of haemoglobin (Hb) in red blood cells. May be conjugated (bound to albumin) or unconjugated (unbound and so able to cross the blood–brain barrier and cause brain damage).

Jaundice: The common term for hyperbilirubinaemia. It can be physiological or pathological.

Phototherapy: Treatment for jaundice, involving placing a neonate under blue fluorescent lights, sometimes called bili-lights.

Conventional phototherapy: Phototherapy given using a single light source (not fibre optic) that is positioned above the neonate.

Fibre optic phototherapy: Phototherapy given using a single light source that comprises a light generator, a fibre optic cable through which the light is carried and a flexible light pad, on which the neonate is placed or it can be wrapped around them.

Metalloporphyrins: Drugs that inhibit heme oxygenase, an enzyme involved in the breakdown of heme (from red blood cells) to bilirubin. By preventing the formation of bilirubin, they have the potential to reduce the level of unconjugated bilirubin.

Multiple phototherapy: Phototherapy that is given using more than one light source simultaneously; for example, two or more conventional units, or a combination of conventional and fibre optic units. Termed 'double' or 'triple' phototherapy given for high levels of bilirubin particularly in pathological jaundice.

Pathological jaundice: Due to a disease process appearing with a rapid onset on day 1 of life.

Physiological jaundice: Due to the normal process of red blood cell breakdown appearing after 3 days of life.

Polycythaemia: An increased concentration of red blood cells in the blood, either through reduction of plasma volume or increase in red cell count.

Prolonged jaundice: Lasting more than 14 days in term neonates and more than 21 days in preterm neonates. May be indicative of a potential and serious condition such as biliary atresia, choledochal cyst, neonatal hepatitis, metabolic disorders (galactosaemia) or a complication of TPN.

Serum bilirubin (SBR): Bile pigment produced by breakdown of haem from red blood cell metabolism which is measured by analyzing blood serum.

Significant hyperbilirubinaemia: An elevation of the serum bilirubin to a level requiring treatment.

Transcutaneous bilirubin: A measurement of bilirubin concentration in the subcutaneous tissue under the skin taken by a non-invasive skin probe/monitor.

Visible jaundice: Jaundice detected by visual inspection.

Jaundice: References

British Committee for Standards in Haematology (2004). Transfusion guidelines for neonates and older children. *British Journal of Haematology.* 124: 433–453.

Ford, K.L. (2010). Detecting neonatal jaundice. *Community Practitioner.* 88 (8): 40–42.

Kumar, P., Chawla, D., and Deorari, A. (2011). Light-emitting diode phototherapy for unconjugated hyperbilirubinaemia in neonates. *Cochrane Database of Systematic Reviews.* Issue 12. Art. No.: CD007969.

Mills, J.F. and Tudehope, D. (2005). Fibre optic phototherapy for neonatal jaundice. *Cochrane Neonatal Group Cochrane Database of Systematic Reviews.* 1: 2007.

National Institute for Clinical Excellence (NICE, 2010). *Neonatal jaundice* http://www.nice.org.uk/nicemedia/live/12986/48679/48679.pdf

National Institute for Clinical Excellence (NICE, 2012). *Neonatal jaundice: Evidence Update March 2012. A summary of selected new evidence relevant to NICE clinical guideline 98 'Neonatal jaundice' (2010).*

O'Conner, M.C., Lease, M.A., and Whalen, B.L. (2013). How to use: Transcutaneous bilirubinometry. *Archives of Disease in Childhood – Education and Practice Edition.* 98 (4): 154–159.

Rennie, J., Burman-Roy, S., and Murphy, M.S. (2010). Guidelines: Neonatal jaundice: Summary of NICE guidance. *BMJ: British Medical Journal.* 340: 2409, 1190–1192.

Sarici, S.U., Koklu, E., and Babacan, O. (2014). Comparison of two transcutaneous bilirubinometers in term and near-term neonates. *Neonatal Network.* 33 (3): 138–142.

Schwartz, H.P., Haberman, B.E., and Ruddy, R.M. (2011). Hyperbilirubinaemia: Current guidelines and emerging therapies. *Pediatric Emergency Care.* 27: 884–889.

Suresh, G., Martin, C.L., and Soll, R. (2003). Metalloporphyrins for treatment of unconjugated hyperbilirubinemia in neonates. *Cochrane Database of Systematic Reviews.* Issue 1. Art. No.: CD004207.

Thayyil, S. and Milligan, D. (2006). Single versus double volume exchange transfusion in jaundiced newborn infants. *Cochrane Database of Systematic Reviews.* Issue 4. Art. No.: CD004592.

Truman, P. (2006). Jaundice in the preterm infant. *Paediatric Nursing.* 18 (5): 20–22.

Turnbull, V. and Petty, J. (2012). Early onset jaundice in the newborn: Understanding the ongoing care of mother and baby. *British Journal of Midwifery.* 20 (9): 540–547.

Tyler, W. and McKiernan, P.J. (2006). Prolonged jaundice in the preterm infant – What to do, when and why. *Current Paediatrics.* 16 (1): 43–50.

Wentworth, S. (2005). Neonatal phototherapy – Today's lights, lamps and devices. *Infant.* 1 (1): 14–19.

Kangaroo care (skin-to-skin)

This chapter covers a key related area to developmental care; that of 'Kangaroo care' otherwise known as skin-to-skin contact.

Early care of healthy neonates in the delivery suite or at home following birth includes the encouragement of early breast feeding and skin-to-skin contact for many reported benefits; namely, improved outcomes (Conde-Agudelo et al., 2011), better neonatal thermal control (Karlsson et al., 2012), reduction of neonatal stress, improved cardio-respiratory stability, decreased crying (Moore et al., 2012), procedural pain relief (Johnston et al., 2014) and facilitation of breast feeding and parental bonding (Lemmen et al., 2013). However, it is a care practice that can be undertaken in any part of the neonatal unit and Box 2.39 outlines the key principles.

Related topics: see also *Developmental care and Pain management* as skin to skin has benefits relating to reduction of stress. *Thermal care* is relevant in relation to where skin-to-skin contact can facilitate thermal balance and prevent heat loss. Finally, this procedure is one of the key areas that can promote bonding and attachment in line with promoting psychological care of parents – see *Psychosocial care of the family*.

Kangaroo or skin-to-skin care can be given to any neonate even those in intensive care, as long as their condition allows, while ensuring family support is given throughout. It is important to consider and offer kangaroo care to *both* parents.

Box 2.39   Principles of skin-to-skin care – FLOW CHART

Preparation

Assess readiness of neonate, parents and neonatal staff/unit

Explain benefits and process to parents. Ensure kangaroo care is part of the developmental care plan

Secure all tubes and lines. Set up position of chair and any support necessary. Get parent(s) into position. Provide blanket and hat for the neonate. Check neonates' vital signs

▽

Transfer

Remove neonate carefully from incubator with another nurse to hold lines or tubes if necessary.

Place upright on parent's chest with legs and arms flexed and head and neck positioned to ensure open airway. The face may be directed towards the parent's face. Keep neonate against the skin but covered over their back with a hat on

▽

Monitoring**

Continue with vital sign monitoring including pulse oximetry

Check temperature regularly according to neonate's gestation and thermal stability

Assess comfort levels

Tube feeding can continue

▽

Transfer back

Move back to incubator when ready/appropriate

Document time of kangaroo care

For a more evidence-based detailed guide to kangaroo care, refer to Ludington-Hoe, et al. (2008)

**If neonate shows signs of instability (apnoea, desaturation, drops in central temperature), kangaroo care may not be appropriate at that time. In addition, contraindications include any neonate with a chest drain, arterial line, on high frequency ventilation or inhaled nitric oxide or one who has been unstable within the last 24 hours.

 Check local guidance for skin-to-skin care policy.

Kangaroo care: Glossary

Kangaroo care: Holding a newborn or neonate using skin-to-skin contact.

Skin-to skin contact: A newborn or older neonate is placed bare-skinned directly onto their mother or father's skin, usually the chest.

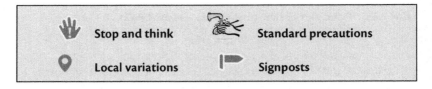

Stop and think

Standard precautions

Local variations

Signposts

Always wash hands when touching or moving a neonate for skin-to-skin contact and advise parents to do the same before handling them.

The space below can be used to record any local variations and practice points specific to your own unit.

Kangaroo care: References

Conde-Agudelo, A., Belizán, J.M., and Diaz-Rosella, J. (2011). Kangaroo mother care to reduce morbidity and mortality in low birthweight infants. *Cochrane Database of Systematic Reviews*. Issue 3. Art. No.: CD002771.

Johnston, C., Campbell-Yeo, M., Fernandes, A., Inglis, D., Streiner, D., and Zee, R. (2014). Skin-to-skin care for procedural pain in neonates. *Cochrane Database of Systematic Reviews*. Issue 1. Art. No.: CD008435.

Karlsson, V., Heinemann, A., Sjörs, G., Nykvist, K.H., and Ågren, J. (2012). Early skin-to-skin care in extremely preterm infants: Thermal balance and care environment. *The Journal of Pediatrics*. 161 (3): 422–426.

Lemmen, D., Fristedt, P., and Lundqvist, A. (2013). Kangaroo care in a neonatal context: Parents' experiences of information and communication of nurse-parents. *The Open Nursing Journal*. 7: 41–48. http://www.ncbi.nlm.nih.gov/pmc/articles/PMC3680980/

Ludington-Hoe, S.M., Morgan, K., and Abouelfettoh, A. (2008). A clinical guideline for implementation of Kangaroo care with premature infants of 30 or more weeks postmenstrual age. *Advances in Neonatal Care*. 8 (3) (Suppl): S3–S23.

Moore, E.R., Anderson, G.C., Bergman, N., and Dowswell, T. (2012). Early skin-to-skin contact for mothers and their healthy newborn infants. *Cochrane Database of Systematic Reviews*. Issue 5. Art. No.: CD003519.

Further reading: kangaroo care

A sound body of theory underpins this topic and the reader may refer to the following selected open access resources to explore this further.

Chui, S. (2010). Effect of early skin-to-skin contact on mother preterm infant interaction through 18 months: Randomized controlled trials. *Journal of International Nursing Studies*. 46 (9): 1168–1180. http://www.ncbi.nlm.nih.gov/pmc/articles/PMC2818078/

Curran, R.L., Genesoni, L., Huertas Ceballos, A., and Tallandini, M.A. (2008). A kangaroo mother care research study: A work in progress.

Infant. 4 (5): 163–165. http://www.neonatal-nursing.co.uk/pdf/inf_023_mer.pdf

Lawn, J.E., Mwansa-Kambafwile, J., Horta, B.L., Barros, F.C., and Cousens, S. (2010). Kangaroo mother care' to prevent neonatal deaths due to preterm birth complications. *Int. J. Epidemiol*. 39 (Suppl 1): i144–i154. doi: 10.1093/ije/dyq031. http://ije.oxfordjournals.org/content/39/suppl_1/i144.full

Levels of dependency

This chapter focuses on the organization of neonatal care in relation to the term 'dependency'.

The Department of Health (UK DoH, 2009) and the British Association of Perinatal Medicine (BAPM, 2011) outline the four levels of dependency within neonatal care – transitional, special, high dependency and intensive care (Table 2.26) – regarding the level of support a neonate requires as well as the recommended staffing levels (nurse: patient ratio) required.

> **Related topics.** See also *The multi-disciplinary team* in relation to discharge planning as a neonate improves, becomes less dependent and lowers their need for clinical support. *Gastrointestinal care and feeding* also summarizes feeding methods in relation to dependency levels in Figure 2.21. Similarly, *Thermal care* outlines methods used to keep neonates warm from intensive through to transitional care in Figure 2.42.

> **A neonate can move in any direction between levels of dependency – for example, from intensive care through to lower dependency when their condition is improving until they go home. Of course, if they become unwell at any point, then they may move back into a higher dependency level.**

Table 2.26   Levels of care (dependencies) – SUMMARY TABLE

Intensive care – one-to-one ratio (nurse to patient)
A neonate receiving any form of mechanical respiratory support via a tracheal tube. Day of surgery, day of death, any day receiving any of the following: presence of an umbilical arterial or venous line, peripheral arterial line, insulin infusion, chest drain, exchange transfusion, therapeutic hypothermia, prostaglandin infusion, replogle tube, epidural catheter, silo for gastroschisis, external ventricular drain

High dependency care – one-to-two ratio (nurse to patient)
Any of the following apply: any day receiving any form of non-invasive respiratory support (e.g. nasal CPAP, BIPAP) and/or any day receiving any of the following: parenteral nutrition, continuous infusion of drugs (except prostaglandin and/or insulin), presence of a central venous or intravenous long line, tracheostomy, urethral or suprapubic catheter, trans-anastomotic tube following oesophageal atresia repair, nasal airway/nasal stent, observation of seizures/cerebral function monitoring, barrier nursing, ventricular tap

---

(continued)

Table 2.26   Continued

Special care – one-to-four ratio (nurse to patient)
Special care is any of the following: oxygen by nasal cannula, feeding by nasogastric, jejenal tube or gastrostomy, continuous physiological monitoring (excluding apnoea monitors only), care of a stoma, presence of IV cannula, phototherapy, special observation of physiological variables at least 4 hourly

Transitional care

General principle: Delivered within a dedicated transitional care ward or within a postnatal ward. In either case the mother must be resident with her neonate and providing care. Care is provided by parents with support from a healthcare professional. Examples include low birth-weight neonates, those who are stable with neonatal abstinence syndrome and those requiring a specific treatment that can be administered on a postnatal ward, such as antibiotics or phototherapy.

Source: Adapted with kind permission from British Association of Perinatal Medicine (BAPM, 2010, 2011)

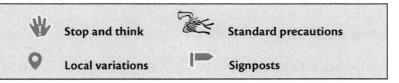

🖐	**Stop and think**		**Standard precautions**
📍	**Local variations**	➤	**Signposts**

📍 **The space below can be used to record any local variations and practice points specific to your own unit.**

Levels of dependency: Glossary

Dependency: The level of support a neonate requires to treat and optimize their condition.

High dependency care: Care provided for those who require highly skilled staff but where the nurse to patient ratio is less than that of intensive care.

Intensive care: Care provided for neonates who are the most unwell or unstable and have the greatest needs

in relation to staff skills and staff to patient ratios.

Special care: Care provided for those who require additional care delivered by the neonatal service but do not require either intensive or high dependency care.

Transitional care: Care received within a postnatal ward or transitional care unit prior to discharge home.

Level of Dependency: References

BAPM. (2010). *Service standards for hospitals providing neonatal care (3rd edition).* http://www.bapm.org/publications/documents/guidelines/BAPM_Standards_Final_Aug2010.pdf

BAPM. (2011). *Categories of care* http://www.bapm.org/publications/documents/guidelines/CatsofcarereportAug11.pdf

UK Department of Health (DoH; 2009). *Toolkit for neonatal services* http://webarchive.nationalarchives.gov.uk/20130107105354/http://www.dh.gov.uk/prod_consum_dh/groups/dh_digitalassets/@dh/@en/@ps/@sta/@perf/documents/digitalasset/dh_108435.pdf

Multi-disciplinary team (MDT)

This chapter covers two related areas; the multi-disciplinary team (MDT) within the neonatal unit and discharge planning outlined in Figure 2.26 and Box 2.40.

Team working is an essential part of effective communication (RCN, 2007). Neonates in the neonatal unit (NNU) need constant monitoring and 24-hour care from a variety of healthcare professionals. Figure 2.26 highlights some of the staff members that a neonate and parent may encounter.

The MDT has a vital role to play in the discharge planning for all neonates with nurses taking a central role in the majority of preparations. The main aim of care at any stage of illness or gestation is for the neonate and family to be discharged home with support where applicable, without the 24 hour care of the neonatal unit. Specific challenges to be achieved prior to discharge are the transition of thermal adaptation, nutritional management and establishment of feeding, and the avoidance of post-discharge problems. Box 2.40 summarizes some of the important factors to consider prior to discharge and shows where the MDT fits within the whole process.

The theme of MDT working is relevant throughout this book since for any aspect of holistic care of the neonate and family, inter-professional communication is essential. This topic is therefore applicable to all chapters. In particular, of course, *Communication* is an essential element of MDT working.

Effective communication and team-working are two vital elements of an MDT that is effective in providing holistic, planned and structured care to a neonate and family (Brown et al., 2003; Barwell et al., 2013; Bayliss-Pratt, 2013).

Figure 2.26 The multi-disciplinary team in neonatal care – DIAGRAM

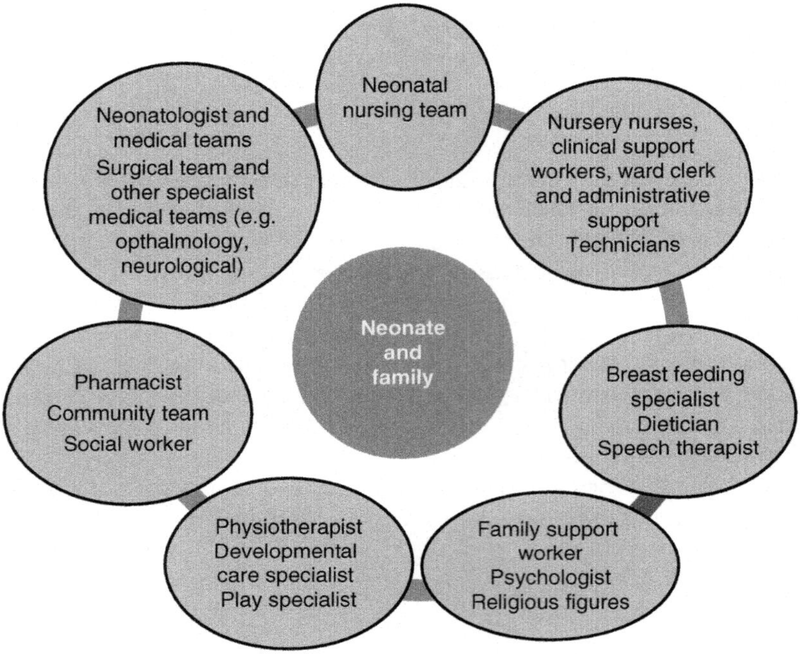

Check local MDT structure and communication / referral processes

Box 2.40 Discharge home – CHECKLIST

Prior to discharge
- Designated staff agree discharge date with parents or persons with parental responsibility
- Start plan a minimum of 48 hours prior to discharge

Parent education
- Administration of medications when required
- Parentcraft/baby cares (e.g. nappy changes, top and tailing, bathing etc.)
- Feeding/making up feeds
- Nasogastric tube feeding where necessary
- Use of car seat
- Basic infant resuscitation (practical demonstration)
- Thermoregulation
- Respiratory syncytial virus (RSV)

(continued)

- Immunizations, if not already received (give national leaflet)
- Prevention of cot death leaflet
- Parent to learn night-time routine by 'rooming in' overnight with their neonate

Parent communication

- Check home and discharge addresses and confirm name of GP with parents
- Complete red book and give to parents
- Give parents copy of discharge summary and allow them time to ask questions after they have read it
- Complete neonatal dataset by date of discharge
- Ensure all follow-up appointments are made (see below)
- Perform and record discharge examination (medical team)

Professional communication

- Complete admission book entries
- Inform:
  o health visitor (HV) of discharge, community midwife if neonate < 10 days old
  o GP, community neonatal or paediatric team as required locally
- Safeguarding issues if applicable need communicating
- Vulnerability criteria checked e.g. mental health issues, social circumstances

Procedures/investigations

- Check newborn blood spot was taken
- Check if newborn blood spot was repeated if neonate was born preterm or for other reasons
- Inform community team of need to repeat newborn blood spot if required
- When immunization (2, 3 and 4 month) not complete in preterm infants, inform GP and health visitor
- Arrange appointment for BCG vaccination if required (see local BCG immunization guideline)
- Complete audiology screening and confirm ophthalmology appointment date if required

Other

- Equipment loan to be organized if applicable
- Home oxygen therapy required? – order oxygen, assessment of home environment, housing arrangements ascertained
- Day of discharge: check medications, weight, all parent information clear

Follow-up appointments with the MDT

Appointments may include:

- Neonatal/paediatric consultant outpatients and/or tertiary consultant outpatients (e.g. surgical)
- Ophthalmology screening
- Audiology referral

(continued)

- Brain scanning
- Physiotherapy
- Dietician
- Community paediatrician
- Child development checks
- Further immunizations (e.g. Palivizumab)
- Planned future admission (e.g. for immunizations, blood taking, wound review)

🅠 Check local guidance for discharge planning procedure.

References: Loughren, 2012; Hall et al., 2013; Jefferies, 2014

🖐 Discharge planning begins at admission and continues throughout a neonate's stay in hospital. It is not only a teaching process but should involve the parents in every aspect of their neonate's care. (Loughren, 2012; Hall et al., 2013; Dellenmark-Blom and Wigert, 2014; Raines, 2014).

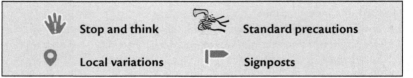

🖐 **Stop and think**   🖐 **Standard precautions**

🅠 **Local variations**   ▶ **Signposts**

🖐 All members of the MDT who care for the neonate and family should be mindful of the importance of standard precautions and the recommended strategies to minimise infection risk. Hand hygiene is a key example of an essential care practice for every team member including the family.

🅠 The space below can be used to record any local variations and practice points specific to your own unit.

The multi-disciplinary team: Glossary

The Multi-disciplinary team in neonatal care: Neonates in the neonatal unit (NNU) need constant monitoring and 24-hour care from a variety of healthcare professionals. Here are some of the staff members that a parent or neonate may encounter.

Administrator: Responsible for a combination of administrative and secretarial roles often providing personal assistant support at meetings and for the lead nurse/NNU consultants.

Advanced Neonatal Nurse Practitioner (ANNP): A registered nurse who has advanced and specialized training in working with premature and sick newborns. He or she can perform many advanced skills/procedures and work at a higher level of decision making.

Breast Feeding specialist: A health professional who supports mothers to breast feed and express, store and handle their breast milk.

Clinical support worker: Health professional who is part of the non-nurse registered workforce who provide clinical support to the team. Healthcare assistants provide one example.

Community neonatal nurse: A neonatal nurse who cares for the neonate and family after discharge in the community/home setting.

Developmental care specialist: A health professional who has received training in the principles of developmental care to advise and support both parents and staff in its application to preterm neonates.

Dietician: A professional who advises and recommends special feeding regimens.

Family Support worker: A health professional who has the primary role to support the parents of neonates during their hospital stay.

Neonatal nurse: Registered nurse who may or may not have completed additional post-qualifying neonatal training. Those who have completed such a course are called 'qualified in specialty' (QIS) and can then progress to higher bands as part of their career development.

Neonatologist: A paediatrician/consultant with advanced training in the care of premature and sick neonates. There may be several neonatologists in the NNU.

Neonatology fellow/registrar: A fully-trained paediatrician who is receiving advanced training in the care of premature and sick neonates and is often the most senior physician in the NNU late at night.

Neonatal senior house officer: A trained doctor who is undertaking a rotation in neonatal care.

Nursery nurse: Part of the non-registered workforce who have completed nursery nurse training at NVQ level and form an integral part of the neonatal nursing team and care.

Occupational therapist: A health professional whose work is based on engagement in meaningful activities of daily life, especially to enable or encourage participation in such activities in spite of impairments or limitations in physical or mental functions. In neonatal care, they aim to improve these functions in the newborn with various interventions to limit any developmental problems caused by neonatal care.

Pharmacist: A professional who is responsible for ensuring correct and safe administration of neonatal drugs and advises on drug indication, dose and availability for all neonates on the NNU.

Physiotherapist: A professional who treats injury or dysfunction with exercises and other physical treatments of the disorder. In the care of the neonate, they may deal with neurological conditions or may be part of the respiratory management of neonates requiring ventilation.

Play specialist: A professional who is trained in the use of age appropriate play interventions and stimulation for children in the hospital setting.

Psychologist: A professional who is an expert in psychology and who can provide emotional support for parents and staff.

Religious figure: A priest, minister, rabbi, imam or other religious advisor, who can provide spiritual support and counselling to help families cope with the stressors of the neonatal unit experience.

Social worker: A professional who is specially trained to help families cope with the social aspects of their neonate's stay in hospital and thereafter. They can help parents deal with financial difficulties and make any special arrangements for the neonate's discharge and follow-up care.

Speech and language therapist: A professional who is trained in speech and language problems, but often works with neonates in NNUs to help assist them with feeding problems.

Technicians: Staff members who are responsible for the upkeep, maintenance and often staff training of equipment required for care delivery in the NNU, for example, ventilators, syringe pumps, blood gas machines.

Ward clerk: Responsible for the running and manning of the front desk dealing with reception and support tasks to the NNU team. An essential member of the team for efficient communication between team members and families and staff.

The multi-disciplinary team: References

Bayliss-Pratt, L. (2013). Training to promote multidisciplinary working. *Nursing Times.* 109 (13): 12–13.

Barwell, J., Arnold, F., and Berry, H. (2013). How interprofessional learning improves care. *Nursing Times.* 109 (21): 14–16.

Brown, M.S., Ohlinger, J., Rusk, C., Delmore, P., and Ittmann, P. (2003). Implementing potentially better practices for multidisciplinary team building: Creating a neonatal intensive care unit culture of collaboration. *Pediatrics, 111* (Suppl. E1): e482–e488.

Dellenmark-Blom, M. and Wigert, H. (2014). Parents' experiences with neonatal home care following initial care in the neonatal intensive care unit: a phenomenological hermeneutical interview study. *Journal of Advanced Nursing.* 70 (3): 575–586.

Hall, E.O., Kronborg, H., Aagaard, H., and Brinchmann, B.S. (2013). The journey towards motherhood after a very preterm birth: Mothers' experiences in hospital and after home-coming. *Journal of Neonatal Nursing.* 19 (3): 109–113.

Jefferies, A.L. (2014). Going home: Facilitating discharge of the preterm infant. *Paediatrics & Child Health.* 19 (1): 31–42.

Loughren, K.J. (2012). Discharge planning in the neonatal intensive care unit. *Journal of Obstetric, Gynecologic, & Neonatal Nursing.* 41: S54.

Raines, D.A. (2014). Preparing for NICU discharge: Mothers' concerns. *Neonatal Network.* 32 (6): 399–403.

Royal College of Nursing and the NHS Institute for Innovation and Improvement (2007). *Developing and Sustaining effective teams.* http://www.rcn.org.uk/__data/ assets/pdf_file/0003/78735/ 003115.pdf

Neurological care and neonatal abstinence syndrome

This chapter covers practice-based tools in relation to the topics of neurological care and neonatal abstinence syndrome.

Neurological care

A healthy neonate will display signs of an intact central nervous system (CNS) such as normal reflexes, behaviour and responses to stimulation. The CNS of the sick and/or preterm neonate, however, is more vulnerable to the effects of hypoxia, infection, trauma or any other event that can potentially damage the developing system (Levene, 2008a; 2008b). This section begins with an overview of the causes of neurological compromise in the neonate. It then turns to some specific neurological conditions in relation to the assessment tools and strategies used in neonatal practice to diagnose or manage them (Boxes 2.41a-c–2.43 and Table 2.27).

> Related topics. See *Assessment* as neurological assessment is part of a holistic approach. *Developmental care* and *Pain management* are also relevant topics as these concern themselves with a vulnerable, immature nervous system, brain and the consequences of care on outcome.

Box 2.41a   Overview of the causes of neurological compromise in the neonate – SUMMARY TABLE

- **Hypoxic-ischaemic encephalopathy*** (HIE): (See Table 2.27) Significant hypoxia during or at birth
- **Haemorrhage**; intra-ventricular (IVH* See Box 2.41c), intra-cerebral, sub-dural, post-haemorrhagic hydrocephalus*
- **Central nervous system infection**; meningitis*, intrauterine (TORCH) infections, other postnatal pathogens (See *Infection* chapter)
- **Compromised blood supply to the brain postnatally**; e.g. perinatal stroke, periventricular leukomalacia (PVL)*
- **Metabolic conditions**; hypoglycaemia, hypo/hypernatraemia, hypocalcaemia, hypomagnesaemia, pyridoxine deficiency
- **Congenital conditions**; Chromosomal and/or congenital brain anomalies (for example, hydrocephalus*, neural tube defects*), neuro-degenerative disorders
- **Drug withdrawal syndromes**; e.g. Neonatal abstinence syndrome
- **Seizures***; (See Box 2.41b)

Note: *Refer to chapter glossary for definitions of conditions

---

Box 2.41b   Neonatal seizure classification – SUMMARY TABLE

All the above conditions outlined in Box 2.41a can cause seizures.

Clinical signs*

- **Subtle**: Eyes staring and/or horizontal deviation. Oral mouthing, chewing, sucking, lip smacking. Limb movement such as swimming, boxing, pedalling. Apnoea, tachycardia and unstable blood pressure are common autonomic signs.
- **Clonic**: Rhythmic jerking, focal (e.g. limbs or one side of body) or multifocal (irregular). **
- **Tonic**: The whole body or one extremity, generalized extension of upper and lower limbs, may be sustained posture of limbs (focal).
- **Myoclonic**: Isolated, rapid jerking,** may be focal (one limb) or multifocal (several parts of the body).

Notes: * Seizure activity should be distinguished from jitteriness which is a normal finding in many neonates. Seizures are not provoked by stimuli, they are predominatly clonic/tonic with altered consciousness and eye deviation and do not cease when limbs are held. Jitteriness however, is stimulus provoked, tremulous in nature without loss of consciousness or eye deviation and stops when the limbs are held.

**Seizures should be also distinguished from benign idiopathic neonatal convulsions: e.g. the 'Fifth day fits' and other benign activity which cease with a good prognosis within a few weeks from birth.

Intraventricular haemorrhage grades

Intraventricular haemorrhage (IVH) is a significant complication of prematurity and so a common condition seen within the neonatal unit. IVH initiates in the fragile germinal matrix, a richly vascularized area lining the ventricles in the developing brain affected by disturbances in the cerebral blood flow (CBF). Papile's grading (Papile et al, 1978) is the most commonly cited tool used to measure the extent of this condition and is depicted overleaf (Ballabh, 2010).

Box 2.41c   Intraventricular haemorrhage (IVH) grades – SUMMARY TABLE

- **Grade I**
  - ○ Restricted to sub-ependymal region/**germinal matrix**. Overall good prognosis
- **Grade II**
  - ○ Extension into **normal** sized ventricles and typically filling less than 50% of the volume of the ventricle. Overall good prognosis
- **Grade III**
  - ○ Extension into **dilated** ventricles – poor outcomes* likely
- **Grade IV**
  - ○ Grade III with **parenchymal (tissue)** haemorrhage. Higher rates of poor outcomes*

Reference: Papile et al (1978)

Additional information

*Poor outcomes include complications such as post-bleed hydrocephalus, damage to the brain tissue leading to long-term developmental delay and increased mortality risk.

Preterm neonates will have a head ultrasound carried out soon after delivery and admission and then regularly thereafter while on the neonatal unit.

 Observe local guidance on agreed classification system for IVH

Gentle handling and caution with care procedures should be considered to safeguard the vulnerable brain and prevent haemodynamic instability which is associated with IVH and PVL (Limperopoulos et al., 2008; Annibale and Rosenkrantz, 2012).

Hypoxic-ischaemic encephalopathy

Hypoxic-ischaemic encephalopathy (HIE), previously known as 'perinatal asphyxia' is characterized by acute or subacute brain injury due to systemic hypoxaemia and/or reduced cerebral blood flow (CBF) before or at birth (Ferriero, 2004; Zanelli, 2013). The most commonly cited framework is the Sarnet Staging system (Sarnet and Sarnet, 1976) which identifies three levels of severity. Table 2.27 below highlights the important areas for assessment in the recognition of HIE.

Table 2.27   Recognizing Hypoxic-Ischaemic Encephalopathy (HIE) – SUMMARY TABLE
Depending on the extent of the hypoxic insult during birth, there will be varying responses and signs in some or all of the following areas:
• Altered level of consciousness
• Muscle tone
• Reflex activity: sucking, Moro, tonic neck, responses to stimulation at birth, eye movements and pupil responses
• Spontaneous respiratory effort and the need for ventilation support
• Heart rate
• Ability to feed
• Presence of seizures
• Duration of signs- these may last for a few days up to weeks depending on whether the hypoxic insult was mild or more severe.
📍   Observe local guidance on agreed classification system for HIE

> 🖐 **The extent of hypoxic damage from HIE influences the care given and the long-term developmental outcome (Perlman, 2004).**

Therapeutic cooling

Evidence supports the use of therapeutic hypothermia for term newborn infants with moderate-to-severe hypoxic ischaemic encephalopathy, as it has been found to reduce the combined outcome of death or long-term neurodevelopmental disability at 18 months (Jacobs et al., 2013; Witt, 2013). The criteria for cooling need to be clear so that neonatal staff understand the process of referral.

> 🖐 **Therapeutic cooling is undertaken in specific neonatal units to which neonates are referred and transferred. However, passive cooling can be commenced in any neonatal unit once referral for 'active' therapeutic cooling is decided and can be done by simple measures such as turning off the incubator temperature, leaving portholes open and leaving only a nappy on the neonate.**

Box 2.42a   Therapeutic cooling criteria – CHECKLIST

(A + B)

A. Neonates >36 weeks gestation with at least one of the following:
- Apgar score of <5 at 10 minutes after birth (See Table 2.2 in *Assessment*)
- Continued need for resuscitation, including endotracheal or mask ventilation, at 10 minutes after birth
- Acidosis within 60 minutes of birth (pH <7)
- Base deficit −16 mmol/l within 60 minutes of birth

Infants who fulfil the A criteria should be assessed for whether they fulfil the B criteria.

B. Moderate-to-severe encephalopathy, consisting of altered state of consciousness (lethargy, stupor or coma) AND at least one of the following:
- Abnormal tone such as hypotonia
- Abnormal reflexes including oculomotor or pupillary abnormalities
- An absent or weak suck
- Clinical seizures,

Cooling should be started within 6 hours (continued for 72 hours)

Source: Used with kind permission from the National Perinatal Epidemiology Unit (NPEU, 2010).
Other useful references: Shah et al. (2007); Azzopardi et al. (2009); British Association of Perinatal Medicine (BAPM, 2010); Jacobs et al. (2013).

Box 2.42b   Therapeutic cooling: nursing overview – FLOW CHART

Preparation

- In a cooling unit, prepare equipment (cooling blanket or bed)
- If in a non-cooling unit, arrange neonatal transfer
- Any unit, start passive cooling and take temperature regularly (every 15 minutes)
- Parental consent

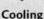

Cooling

- Body is cooled to 33–34°C (no lower than 33°C)
- Central/rectal temperature via probe is taken continually

(continued)

- Cerebral function monitoring is undertaken during cooling along with all vital signs
- Observe heart rate baseline which may be lower than previous readings
- Ensure CO_2 does not drop below 5kPa on blood gas analysis (cooling can cause alkalosis)
- Coagulation is checked
- Fluids restricted
- Observe for pain and discomfort. Morphine given and sedation if required
- Assess tissue viability and observe for possible fat necrosis

▽
Re-warming

- Re-warm 0.5 degrees every 2 hours as a suggested rate
- When central temperature is at an agreed value, switch cooling off
- Observe carefully during re-warming (blood pressure may drop)
- Follow-up, scans and referral to the central register

 Check local guidance on agreed cooling policy if applicable or that relating to referral for cooling
Source: Used with kind permission from the National Perinatal Epidemiology Unit (NPEU, 2010).

Re-warming should be done carefully and slowly avoiding large, sudden increases in the central temperature.

Cerebral function monitoring

Amplitude integrated electroencephalogram (aEEG) monitoring allows the ability to view the activity of the brain over long periods of time at the bedside. Neonates considered for cerebral function monitoring (CFM) include: any neonate who has likely HIE, is receiving therapeutic cooling for HIE, is suspected or at high risk of having seizures and/or abnormal movements and neonates with unexplained neurological signs.

Box 2.43   Cerebral function monitoring – CHECKLIST

Application

- Sensor/electrode application on the scalp; see manufacturer's instructions
- Hydrogel or low impedance needle electrodes. Hydrogel electrodes are preferable to avoid discomfort and they adhere better in warm conditions. Water can be used to rehydrate hydrogel electrodes
- Electrodes must be a minimum of 2 mm apart for correct tracing to be recorded. Low impedance is necessary for a 'clean' trace while the presence of impedance may artificially interfere with the trace
- Care should be taken to prevent electrodes from becoming accidentally dislodged

Recording of events

- Nursing care and procedures undertaken in the care of the neonate receiving cerebral function monitoring (CFM) should be recorded. This is used when interpreting the data

Ongoing assessment

- Observe/assess clinical signs displayed by the neonate during CFM and document/report accordingly, for example, vital signs, abnormal movement and tone

Check local guidance on agreed procedures for performing CFM.

Interpretation of CFM data is carried out by a health professional who is trained in classifying aEEG traces and experienced with the expected patterns exhibited, both normal and abnormal (ter Horst et al., 2006; Hellström-Westas et al., 2006).

  Stop and think   **Standard precautions**

  Local variations   **Signposts**

The importance of preventing infection in relation to the neonate's vulnerable brain and neurological system should be emphasised.

The space below can be used to record any local variations and practice points specific to your own unit.

Neurological Care: Glossary

Cerebral function monitoring (CFM): Provides information on electrical activity of the brain and information on duration, intensity and frequency of neonatal seizures.

Fat necrosis: An uncommon disorder characterized by firm, red nodules and plaques over areas of the body, a documented potential complication of therapeutic cooling in the neonate.

Hydrocephalus: An abnormal increase in the amount of cerebrospinal fluid within the cerebral ventricles of the brain.

Hypoxic ischaemic encephalopathy (HIE): A condition characterized by clinical and laboratory evidence of acute or sub-acute brain injury due to lack of oxygen before or during birth.

Intraventricular haemorrhage (IVH): IVH refers to bleeding within the ventricles of the brain and is most common in the smallest premature neonates.

Jitteriness: Tremors that represent excited neuromuscular activity of newborns. It is transient and harmless. It is often confused with neonatal seizure activity.

LP (lumbar puncture or spinal tap): Insertion of a hollow needle between the vertebrae of the lower back to withdraw cerebrospinal fluid for analysis. May be part of a full septic screen.

Meningitis: Inflammation of the meninges, caused by viral or bacterial infection.

Neural tube defect: Birth defect of the brain or spinal cord occuring in the first month of pregnancy. The two most common are myelomeningocele (spina bifida) where the fetal spinal cord does not close completely; and anencephaly where there is an absence of a major portion of the brain.

Passive cooling: The act of reducing the central body temperature of a neonate by passive (non-invasive) means such as turning off the incubator and reducing layers around the body.

Periventricular leukomalacia (PVL) – A form of brain injury, characterized by the necrosis of white matter near the lateral ventricles (periventricular area) of the brain caused by compromised blood perfusion. Premature neonates are at the greatest risk of the disorder. Can lead to cerebral palsy.

Seizure: A period of uncontrolled electrical impulses in the brain, resulting from a variety of causes. Also termed 'fit' or 'convulsion'. The different types in the neonatal period include subtle, tonic, clonic, myoclonic seizures and benign idiopathic convulsions.

Therapeutic cooling: Treatment for moderate-to-severe HIE where the body is cooled by application of a mattress or wrap for a given period according to specific criteria.

Neurological care: References

Annibale, D.J. and Rosenkrantz, T. (2012). Periventricular hemorrhage-intraventricular hemorrhage. http://emedicine.medscape.com/article/976654-overview.

Azzopardi, D.V., Strohm, B., Edwards, A.D., Dyet, L., Halliday, H.L., Juszczak, E., Kapellou, O., Levene, M., Marlow, N., Porter, E., Thoresen, M., Whitelaw, A., and Brocklehurst, P. (2009). TOBY study group. Moderate hypothermia to treat perinatal asphyxial encephalopathy. *N Engl J Med*. 361 (14): 1349–1358.

Ballabh, P. (2010). Intraventricular hemorrhage in premature infants: mechanism of disease. *Pediatric Research*. 67 (1): 1–8.

British Association of Perinatal Medicine (2010). Position statement on therapeutic cooling for neonatal encephalopathy. http://www.bapm. org/publications/documents/ guidelines/Position_Statement_ Therapeutic_Cooling_Neonatal_ Encephalopathy_July%202010.pdf.

Ferriero, D.M. (2004). Neonatal brain injury. *N Engl J Med*. 351 (19):1985–1995.

Jacobs, S.E., Berg, M., Hunt, R., Tarnow-Mordi, W.O., Inder, T.E., and Davis, P.G. (2013). Cooling for newborns with hypoxic ischaemic encephalopathy. *Cochrane Database of Systematic Reviews*. Issue 1. Art. No.: CD003311.

Hellström-Westas, L., Rosén, I., de Vries, L.S., and Greisen, G. (2006). Amplitude-integrated EEG classification and interpretation in preterm and term infants. *Neoreviews*. 7: e76–e87.

Levene, M. (2008a). Recognition and management of neonatal seizures. *Paediatrics and Child Health*. 18 (4):178–182.

Levene M, Tudehope D, and Sinha S. (2008b). Neurological disorders. In: *Essential Neonatal Medicine*. Oxford: Blackwell Publishing.

Limperopoulos, C., Gauvreau, K.K., O'Leary, H., Moore, M., Bassan, H.,

Eichenwald, E.C., and du Plessis, A.J. (2008). Cerebral hemodynamic changes during intensive care of preterm infants. *Pediatrics*. 122 (5): e1006–e1013.

NPEU. (2010). *UK TOBY cooling register clinicians handbook*. https://www. npeu.ox.ac.uk/downloads/files/ tobyregister/Register-Clinicans-Handbook1-v4-07-06-10.pdf.

Papile LA, Burstein J, Burstein R, Koffler H. (1987). Incidence and evolution of subependymal and intraventricular hemorrhage: A study of infants with birth weight less than 1,500 gm. *J Pediatrics*. 92, 529–34.

Perlman, J.M. (2004). Brain injury in the term infant. *Semin Perinatol*. 28 (6): 415–424.

Sarnat HB, Sarnat MS. (1976). Neonatal encephalopathy following fetal distress: A clinical and electroencephalographic study. *JAMA Neurology (formerly Archives of Neurology)*. 33(10): 696–705.

ter Horst, H.J., Sommer, C., Bergman, K.A., Fock, J.M., van Weerden, T.W., and Bos, A.F. (2006). Prognostic significance of amplitude-integrated EEG during the first 72 hours after birth in severely asphyxiated neonates. *Pediatric Research*. 55 (6): 1026–1033.

Witt, C. (2013). Neuroprotection in the NICU. *Advances in Neonatal Care*. 13

Zanelli, S.A. (2013). Hypoxic-ischemic encephalopathy. http:// emedicine.medscape.com/ article/973501-overview.

Neonatal abstinence syndrome

Neonates born to drug addicted mothers may become dependent on those drugs themselves during pregnancy and then withdraw from that drug after birth. These newborns are said to have neonatal abstinence syndrome (NAS). NAS develops in between 30–80% of all newborns exposed to narcotics *in utero* (Johnson et al., 2003a, 2003b, Jackson, 2006). Although NAS is more typically seen in opiate withdrawal, similar symptoms are seen when withdrawing from benzodiazepines, barbiturates and alcohol (Lall, 2008).

Several abstinence scoring systems can assist nurses and physicians in assessing the severity of NAS withdrawal and providing appropriate therapy (Burgos and Burke, 2009). Box 2.44 outlines an overview of the common features of an assessment tool for NAS used to identify the extent to which a neonate is withdrawing from the passive effects of drugs. Finally, any simple and effective nursing intervention used may help to reduce stress for these vulnerable neonates and their families (Jansson and Velez, 2012).

Related topics. See *Developmental care* and *Environmental care* as these topics concern themselves with care aiming to reduce stress based on behavioural cues.

Assessing the neonate for the presence of NAS or deciding whether to start treatment is open to interpretation due to the subjective nature of assessing neonatal behaviour consistently by different practitioners and at varying times of the day. Attempts should be made to increase objectivity by measures such as providing consistency of allocated nurses if possible and timing of scores.

Box 2.44 Assessing the neonate for neonatal abstinence syndrome (NAS) – CHECKLIST

Neurological features	Gastrointestinal features
Tremors	Uncoordinated sucking
Irritability (excessive crying)	Constant sucking
Increased wakefulness	Increased demand for feeds / hungry
High-pitched crying	Vomiting
Increased muscle tone	Diarrhoea
Hyperactive deep tendon reflexes	Poor weight gain
Exaggerated moro reflex	Potential dehydration
Seizures	
Frequent yawning and sneezing	

Autonomic signs

Mottling
Fever / temperature instability
Increased sweating
Nasal stuffiness / snuffly
Mild elevations in respiratory rate and blood pressure

Scoring: Key points

- Various versions of tools exist but most are based on an original tool by Finnegan and Kaltenbach (1992). Refer to local policy for specific tool in use
- Whatever tool is used however, there are some common elements
- Scoring tools list symptoms that are most frequently observed in NAS
- Each symptom and its associated degree of severity are assigned a score and the total abstinence score is given (Hudak et al, 2012)
- The first abstinence score on admission should be recorded as a baseline score
- Following the baseline score, scoring is done at intervals decided and agreed according to the individual neonate's symptoms, to determine whether treatment is required
- In a term neonate, scoring should be performed after a feed, before they fall asleep. A crying neonate should be soothed and quietened before assessing muscle tone, moro reflex and respiratory rate. Modification may be required for preterm neonates
- Multiple drug misuse alters the pattern of withdrawal (Johnson et al, 2003a)
- The optimal threshold score for starting pharmacologic therapy for NAS is also subject to local unit policy

Check local guidance for NAS scoring

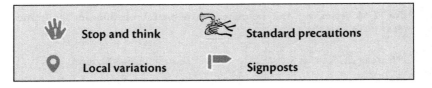

🖐 Stop and think	Standard precautions
📍 Local variations	▶ Signposts

📍 **The space below can be used to record any local variations and practice points specific to your own unit.**

Neonatal abstinence syndrome: Glossary

Illicit drugs: Drugs that are taken for recreational purposes that include heroin, cocaine and marijuana.

Fetal alcohol syndrome: A congenital syndrome associated with excessive consumption of alcohol by the mother during pregnancy, characterized by intellectual and physical developmental delay and dysmorphic features in the neonate, particularly of the skull and face.

Neonatal abstinence syndrome (NAS): A collection of signs and symptoms caused by drug withdrawal in the neonate following the sudden cessation of these drugs at birth, on which the growing fetus has become dependent during pregnancy.

Withdrawal: Drug withdrawal is the group of symptoms that occur upon the abrupt discontinuation or decrease in intake of medications on which the body has become dependent.

Neonatal abstinence syndrome: References

Burgos, A.E. and Burke, B.L. (2009). Neonatal abstinence syndrome. *NeoReviews*. 10 (5): e222–e229.

Finnegan, L.P. and Kaltenbach, K. (1992). Neonatal abstinence syndrome. In: R.A. Hoekelman, S.B. Friedman, N. Nelson, and H.M. Seidel (eds), Primary Pediatric care. (2nd ed). St Louis: C V Mosby.

Hudak, M.L., Tan, R.C., Frattarelli, D.A., Galinkin, J.L., Green, T.P., Neville, K.A., and Watterberg, K.L. (2012). Neonatal drug withdrawal. *Pediatrics*. 129 (2): e540–e560. http://pediatrics. aappublications.org/content/129/2/ e540.short.

Jackson, L. (2006). Handling drug misuse in the neonatal unit. *Infant*. 2 (2): 64–67.

Johnson, K., Gerada, C., and Greenough, A. (2003a). Substance misuse during pregnancy. *The British Journal of Psychiatry*. 183: 187–189. doi: 10.1192/02-346.

Johnson, K., Gerada, C., and Greenough, A. (2003b). Treatment of neonatal abstinence syndrome. *Archives of Disease in Childhood*. 88: F2–5.

Jansson, L.M. and Velez, M. (2012). Neonatal abstinence syndrome. *Current Opinion in Pediatrics*. 24 (2): 252–258.

Lall, A. (2008). Neonatal abstinence syndrome. *British Journal of Midwifery*. 16 (4): 220–223.

Oxygen therapy

This chapter addresses oxygen therapy which is the therapeutic administration of oxygen for the treatment or prevention of hypoxaemia (low blood oxygen levels) or hypoxia (inadequate oxygen at the cellular level).

The goal of oxygen therapy is to achieve adequate delivery of oxygen to the tissue without creating oxygen toxicity (Askie, 2013). A failure to maintain adequate blood oxygen levels can result in progressive deterioration. Figure 2.27, Box 2.45 and Tables 2.28 and 2.29 focus on three important areas: methods of oxygen administration, oxygen monitoring methods and understanding parameters and limits.

> Related areas. Oxygen therapy is an essential area of neonatal ventilation practice and links closely with *Airway* and *Breathing*. Also very important in line with assessment, is oxygenation status along with all other vital signs, so refer also to *Assessment*.

Oxygen administration

The administration of oxygen to neonates requires the selection of an oxygen delivery system that suits the weight, age and the clinical need of the neonate (Fallon, 2012).

> **Neonates including those who require resuscitation should be started in air and then oxygen delivered *according to need* and monitoring values. Once given, it should be weaned as soon as possible. Remember oxygen is a drug with potential risks.**

Figure 2.27 Oxygen therapy overview – DIAGRAM

Facial

For short-term administration only, for example, during resuscitation at birth when required, administered with a bag-valve-mask (BVM) or t-piece (see *Breathing*).

With BVM, quantity delivered is not known. With a t-piece, use an air/oxygen blender.

Always start resuscitation in air and give oxygen according to saturation readings.

Ambient

Into the incubator for up to a 30% oxygen requirement. The incubator will display the % delivered. No need to humidify if <30%. If requirement increases >30% consider head-box and humidify (Fallon, 2012).

Head-box. For 30–50% oxygen, humidify gases. If oxygen requirement increases above 50–60%, consider CPAP (depending also on blood gases and other assessment criteria). Remember to check the % delivered with an oxygen analyzer which should be calibrated to zero.

Neonatal oxygen therapy

High-flow nasal cannula oxygen

Delivery of blended oxygen and air at flow rates of >1 l/min (1–8) (Lawn, 2007; Wilkinson et al., 2011) e.g. via the Vapotherm® device, a thermally controlled humidification system (at 95% or greater relative humidity) that flushes nasopharyngeal dead space. Temperature setting must be 37°C when flow rates >4 l/min and 34–35°C with flow rates <4 l/min. Change water regularly according to local guidelines.

Low-flow nasal cannula oxygen

For low-flow oxygen <1 l/min. The cannula is connected to a wall oxygen connection via a flow meter. Can be humidified if necessary (depending on flow). Read from the centre of the ball in the flow meter; document and record volume being delivered. Low-flow oxygen is necessary for home oxygen therapy.

 Check local guidance and policy on oxygen administration

Box 2.45   Nasal cannula oxygen: additional practice points – CHECKLIST

- Choose appropriate prong size (small or medium). Prongs should fit snugly in the nostrils but there should not be a complete seal
- Secure the cannula – tape it to the face using recommended method agreed locally
- Observe and document vital signs, particularly respiratory pattern and oxygen saturation
- Check for pressure sores on the nares or around the base of nose and cheeks
- Check that the cannula is clear and not blocked with mucous or dirt. Change cannula once a week or more frequently if necessary
- Oxygen requirement is set as required – low flow is <1 l/min and high flow is >1 l/min. 👉 See Figure 2.27

📍 Check local guidance and policy on nasal cannula use

🖐 **A neonate receiving oxygen via any means should be monitored by pulse oximetry in order to assess the efficacy of the therapy and to guide quantity.**

Monitoring oxygenation

As well as monitoring how much is being delivered as above (i.e. in percentages, litres/minute), we must also monitor the actual oxygen levels of the neonate. There are various ways to monitor oxygenation of a neonate receiving respiratory support and oxygen therapy.

Table 2.28   Methods of monitoring oxygen – SUMMARY TABLE

Method	How does it work?	Considerations
Arterial blood	Measures actual tissue oxygen as a partial pressure (kPa or mmHg) via invasive means through aspiration of blood from an in-dwelling arterial line for blood gas analysis	Invasive but is the most accurate measurement of tissue oxygenation
Oxygen saturation (SpO$_2$) via pulse oximetry (Figure 2.28)	Measures the absorption of red and infrared light by pulsatile blood. The relative absorption of light by oxyhaemoglobin and deoxyhaemoglobin is processed by the device and an oxygen saturation level is reported. The result is a continuous measurement of oxyhaemoglobin (%)	Change probe site regularly (at least 4 hourly) to avoid pressure on the skin. Ensure pulsatile trace
Transcutaneous oxygen (TcPO$_2$)	A heated probe applied to the skin measures the 'arterialized' partial pressure values (through the skin) of the underlying capillaries reflecting tissue oxygenation in kPa. This method can also monitor transcutaneous CO$_2$	Calibration is required at each site change (2–4 hourly) to prevent any skin damage
Pre- and post-ductal PaO$_2$ or SpO$_2$ monitoring	Pulse oximetry or blood analysis from the upper (pre-ductal via right hand) and lower/umbilical (post-ductal) body can help identify a right-to-left shunt occurring through the ductus arteriosus Hyperoxia test: principle – due to the right-to-left shunting, placing the neonate in 100% oxygen will not increase arterial saturation. A significant increase in SaO$_2$ means pulmonary disease is likely, but if SaO$_2$ is insignificant or unchanged, a cardiac cause or PPHN is likely	Typically, a difference in upper limbs pre- and post-ductal measurements suggests a right-to-left shunt and a pre- to post-ductal PaO$_2$ gradient can occur in PPHN and/or coarctation of the aorta NB. PPHN is Persistent Pulmonary Hypertension of the Newborn
Oxygenation index (OI)	A calculated value to determine a neonate's oxygen demand and associated level of oxygenation. $$OI = \frac{MAP\ (cm\ H_2O) \times FiO_2 \times 100}{PaO_2\ (mmHg)}$$ Mathur and Seth (2003)	Used as criteria for iNO and/or extra corporeal membrane oxygenation (ECMO) in the very sick newborn

📍 Check local guidance and policy on oxygen monitoring

🖐 **Monitoring of both oxygen delivery and the levels in the blood and tissues is essential to guard against the risk of too little or too much oxygen, both of which have related physiological effects.**

Figure 2.28 Oxygen saturation probe

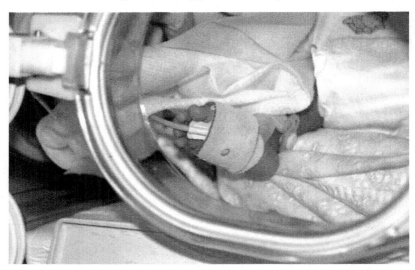

Oxygen monitoring parameters and limits

SpO$_2$ targeting is challenging in preterm infants receiving respiratory support (Askie, 2013) with a high proportion of time spent outside the target range and frequent prolonged hypoxic and hyperoxic episodes (Lim et al., 2014). Targets vary depending on gestation and age (Cherian et al., 2014).

> **Setting appropriate upper and lower limits for oxygen monitoring should be done in line with age, gestation and whether oxygen or air is being required. For example, one can be more liberal with the set limits if a neonate is no longer at risk of retinopathy of prematurity (ROP) and/or once he/she is in air.**

Table 2.29   Oxygen monitoring parameters and limits – SUMMARY TABLE
Arterial Blood – Taken from blood gas analysis. 6.5–10 kPa (neonatal)
Transcutaneous – As for blood gas. 6.5–10 kPa (preterm)/6.5–12 (term)
Oxygen saturations • At birth: Resuscitation Council (2013) state- SaO$_2$ (pre-ductal) in the 1st 10 minutes of life as follows: 2 min 60%, 3 min 70%, 4 min 80%, 5 min 85% and 10 min 90%.

(continued)

Table 2.29   Continued

- After 10 minutes of life: Keep limits 90–95% (subject to local variations) for preterm neonates requiring oxygen before their eyes have vascularized fully.
- For preterm neonates in air or free of the risk of retinopathy of prematurity (ROP), the upper limit can be set higher.
- Keep limits 95–100% in term neonates and those that have pulmonary hypertension.

Check local guidance and policy on setting oxygen monitoring alarm limits

References: SUPPORT Study group, 2010; Bashambu et al., 2012; Lui et al., 2012; Stenson et al; 2013; Lim et al., 2014; Stokowski, 2014.

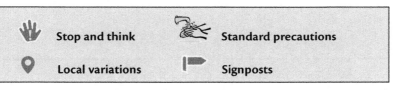

| | Stop and think | | Standard precautions |
| | Local variations | | Signposts |

Ensure standard precautions are maintained in relation to the cleaning of any equipment and adjuncts used to administer oxygen. This is particularly important if oxygen is humidified as a moist environment favours pathogen growth.

The space below can be used to record any local variations and practice points specific to your own unit.

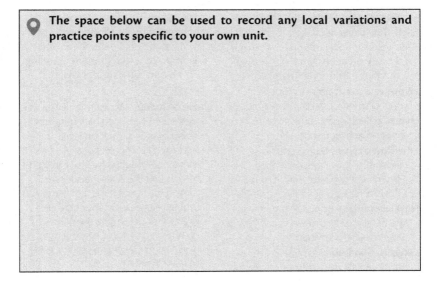

Oxygen therapy: Glossary

Ambient: Relating to the immediate surroundings.

Head-box: Perspex, clear box placed over a neonate's head into which oxygen is delivered to provide immediate ambient oxygen around the face.

High-flow oxygen: Oxygen that is delivered at flow rates higher than 1 l/minute for a neonate usually through a machine called a Vapotherm®.

Hypoxaemia: An abnormally low concentration of oxygen in the blood.

Hypoxia: Deficiency in the amount of oxygen reaching the tissues.

Low-flow oxygen: Oxygen that is delivered at flow rates lower than 1 l/min for a neonate. Administered via a flow meter through a nasal cannula.

Nasal cannula: Soft plastic tubing with fine nasal prongs that delivers a flow of oxygen into the nostrils.

Oxygenation index: An assessment of how much oxygen diffuses across the membranes of the lungs and into the blood.

Oxygen dissociation curve: Plots the proportion of haemoglobin in its saturated form on the vertical axis against the prevailing oxygen tension on the horizontal axis. The oxyhaemoglobin dissociation curve is an important tool for understanding how blood carries and releases oxygen.

Pulse oximeter: Monitoring device that uses a light sensor to help determine blood oxygen saturation levels expressed as a percentage. Used to measure pre-ductal (before the blood has crossed the ductus arteriosus) oxygen saturation (SpO_2) of the blood during resuscitation and thereafter, essential to determine the need for commencing and/or continuing oxygen and gauging necessary levels to administer if necessary.

Transcutaneous oxygen (TcPO$_2$): A measurement of oxygen diffused from capillaries measured through the epidermis.

Transcutaneous monitor: Measures oxygen and carbon dioxide in the blood continuously by the use of a skin probe.

> The Glossaries for *Assessment* and *Breathing* are also relevant for this topic.

Oxygen therapy: References

Askie, L.M. (2013). Optimal oxygen saturations in preterm infants: A moving target. *Current Opinion Pediatrics.* 25 (2):188–192. doi: 10.1097/MOP.0b013e32835e2c00.

Bashambu, M.T., Bhola, M., and Walsh, M. (2012). Evidence for oxygen use in preterm infants. *Acta Paediatrica Suppl.* 101 (464): 29–33. doi:10.1111/j.1651-2227.2011.02548.x.

Cherian, S., Morris, I., Evans, J., and Kotecha, S. (2014). Oxygen therapy in preterm infants. *Paediatric Respiratory Reviews.*15 (2): 135–141.

Fallon, A. (2012). Fact sheet oxygen therapy. *Journal of Neonatal Nursing.* 18 (6): 198–200.

Lawn, C. (2007). High flow humidified oxygen therapy for neonates requiring respiratory support. *Infant.* 3 (3): 105–108. http://www.neonatal-nursing.co.uk/pdf/inf_015_hdd.pdf

Lim, K., Wheeler, K.I., Gale, T.J., Jackson, H.D., Kihlstrand, J.F., Sand, C., and Dargaville, P.A. (2014). Oxygen saturation targeting in preterm infants receiving continuous positive airway pressure. *The Journal of Pediatrics.* 164 (4): 730–736.

Lui, K., Foster, J.P., Davis, P.G., Ching, S.K., Oei, J.L., and Osborn, D.A. (2012). Higher versus lower oxygen concentrations titrated to target oxygen saturations during resuscitation of preterm infants at birth (Protocol).

Cochrane Database of Systematic Reviews. Issue 11. Art. No.: CD010239.

Mathur, N.B. and Seth, A. (2003). Oxygen therapy; Chapter 6. In Gupte, S. (ed.) *Recent Advances in Pediatrics: Special edition Volume 12 – Neonatal Emergencies.* Daryaganj: Jaypee Bro publication.

Stenson, B.J., Tarnow-Mordi, W.O., Darlow, B.A., Simes, J., Juszczak, E., Askie, L., and Brocklehurst, P. (2013). BOOST II United Kingdom collaborative group, BOOST II Australia collaborative group, BOOST II New Zealand collaborative group. Oxygen saturation and outcomes in preterm infants. *The New England Journal of Medicine.* 368 (22): 2094–2104.

Stokowski, L.A. (2014). *Oxygen saturation in preterm infants: Hitting the target.* http://www.medscape.com/viewarticle/820049_3.

SUPPORT Study Group of the Eunice Kennedy Shriver NICHD Neonatal Research Network (2010). Target ranges of oxygen saturation in extremely preterm infants. *The New England Journal of Medicine.* 362 (21): 1959.

Wilkinson, D., Andersen, C., O'Donnell, C.P.F., and De Paoli, A.G. (2011). High flow nasal cannula for respiratory support in preterm infants. *Cochrane Database of Systematic Reviews.* Issue 5. Art. No.: CD006405. DOI: 10.1002/14651858. CD006405.pub2.

Psychosocial care of the family and pain management

This chapter covers the following two topics under 'P'; Psychosocial care of the family and Pain management.

Parents and family centred care principles

Admission to the neonatal unit has significant psychosocial implications for parents. There are a number of family-centred interventions that nurses can deliver that help reduce the stress experienced by parents in the neonatal unit (Chertok et al., 2014). Those elements relating to emotional, psychosocial and family-centred care are detailed below in Table 2.30. Specific elements of this overarching topic have been drawn out to form Figures 2.29–2.31b; namely, a; bonding and attachment, b; partnership and empowerment and c; recognizing diversity.

This section then continues to include ethical decision making and end of life care in Box 2.46 and Figures 2.31c–d . The key points covered in this section contain many common, interconnecting principles that are fundamental to the optimum psychosocial support of the family in the neonatal unit.

> Related topics. See also *Developmental care* and *Communication* for important links with family-centred care and the need to consider the psychosocial needs of the family during a neonate's stay in the neonatal unit.

Table 2.30   Family-centred care principles – SUMMARY TABLE

Charter principle (BLISS, 2011)	How
Neonates should be treated as an individual and with dignity, respecting their social, developmental and emotional needs, as well as their clinical needs. This includes respecting the neonate and family's right to privacy and time to make attachments	✓ Assess the family's needs on admission (Mundy, 2010) ✓ Respect the neonate and parents' right to dignity and privacy ✓ Care is timed and paced to minimize stress, avoid pain and conserve energy ✓ Parents are supported in providing gentle comforting touch that is responsive to their neonate's behavioural cues. This can promote bonding and attachment. (⟹ See Figure 2.29 and 2.31a)

(continued)

Table 2.30   Continued

Charter principle	How
Neonatal care decisions are based on the neonates' best interests, with parents actively involved in their neonate's care and supported in the decision-making process	✓ The whole family is included in planning – both parents and siblings (Feeley et al., 2013) in partnership with staff. (▮➡ See Figure 2.31a) ✓ Care plans are documented with parents ✓ Psychological and social aspects of care are recognized especially at critical times, for example, when receiving sensitive news and at end of life (Robertson et al., 2011) ✓ Sensitive news should be given by appropriately trained staff and in a private environment where support is immediately available (Kendall and Guo, 2008; Branchett and Stretton, 2012)
Neonates receive the nationally recommended level of care in the nearest specialist unit to the family home	✓ The neonatal unit is appropriately staffed to deliver the required level of care ✓ Staff adopt a multi-disciplinary approach to care to best meet the neonate's and family's clinical, psychosocial and developmental needs ✓ Where possible, both mother and neonate are cared for in the same hospital and neonatal unit as close to home as the neonate's condition allows
Parents are informed, guided and supported, so they understand their neonate's care processes and feel confident in caring for them (Nicholas et al., 2014)	✓ Take time to inform parents and provide written information (in a range of formats and languages) (Merritt, 2013). ✓ Consider cultural observances and preferences. (▮➡ See Figure 2.31b) ✓ Attention is paid to groups where English is not the first language (Reitmanova and Gustafson, 2008). ✓ All parents are adequately introduced to facilities, routines, staff and equipment on admission ✓ Inform parents on how they can help to care for their neonate while on the unit and in preparation for discharge (Lee et al., 2014)

(continued)

Table 2.30   Continued

Charter principle	How
	✓ Safe and private facilities are available to parents, making visiting and staying as comfortable as possible (Redshaw and Hamilton, 2010). Rooms need to be suitable with bed etc. ✓ Parents are made aware of national and local support networks and sources of information on the care of their neonates ✓ Consistent and clear information – covering clinical conditions, tests, treatment, risks and outcomes, and practical support – is provided to parents ✓ Daily cares: parents are supported to participate in their neonate's daily routine (Lee et al., 2014)

Source: Based on selected principles from the BLISS Baby Charter (2nd edition, 2011) and NICE (2010) Care Standards. Refer to these documents for full guidance.

Parents of neonates receiving specialist neonatal care should be encouraged and supported to be involved in planning and providing care and regular communication with clinical staff should occur throughout the care pathway (NICE, 2010).

Figure 2.29 Promoting attachment and bonding – DIAGRAM

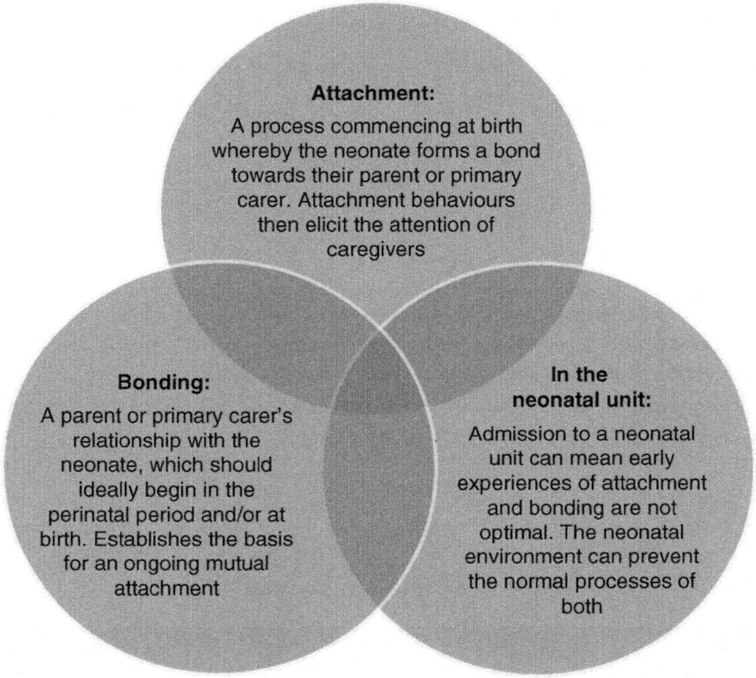

Attachment:
A process commencing at birth whereby the neonate forms a bond towards their parent or primary carer. Attachment behaviours then elicit the attention of caregivers

Bonding:
A parent or primary carer's relationship with the neonate, which should ideally begin in the perinatal period and/or at birth. Establishes the basis for an ongoing mutual attachment

In the neonatal unit:
Admission to a neonatal unit can mean early experiences of attachment and bonding are not optimal. The neonatal environment can prevent the normal processes of both

▽
Strategies to enhance bonding and attachment

- Facilitation of *early* contact between newborn baby and parent(s) is preferred to support the beginning of the attachment process
- Ensure on admission that parents' needs are assessed so that any risk factors can be identified preventing attachment and bonding
- Encourage frequent, regular visits to the neonatal unit thereafter, allowing flexibility and including all family members
- Build supportive relationships with parents as soon as possible ensuring sensitivity to needs and individual requirements
- Encourage active involvement in care as tolerated by the neonate, when the family feel they are ready to participate. (▐➤ See Figure 2.31a)
- Encourage parents/family to watch, touch, hold hands with and talk to their neonate despite any barriers imposed by the neonatal environment (▐➤ see Figure 2.30)

(continued)

- Encourage and support the neonate's mother to express breast milk
- Provide environment for skin-to-skin contact between neonate and parents
- Employ strategies to increase the closeness between neonate and family, such as photographs, diaries, keepsakes, religious symbols in the incubator

Supporting parents to bond with their neonate is an essential aspect of family-centred nursing care in the neonatal unit. It has been shown to improve psychological outcomes for neonate as well as providing positive memories and experiences for the parents (Prior and Glaser, 2006; NHS Health Scotland and CHAS, 2012).

Figure 2.30 Neonate and adult hand

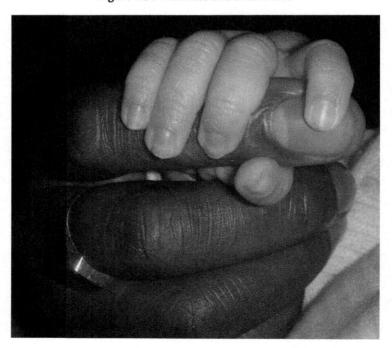

Figure 2.31a Partnership and negotiation – DIAGRAM

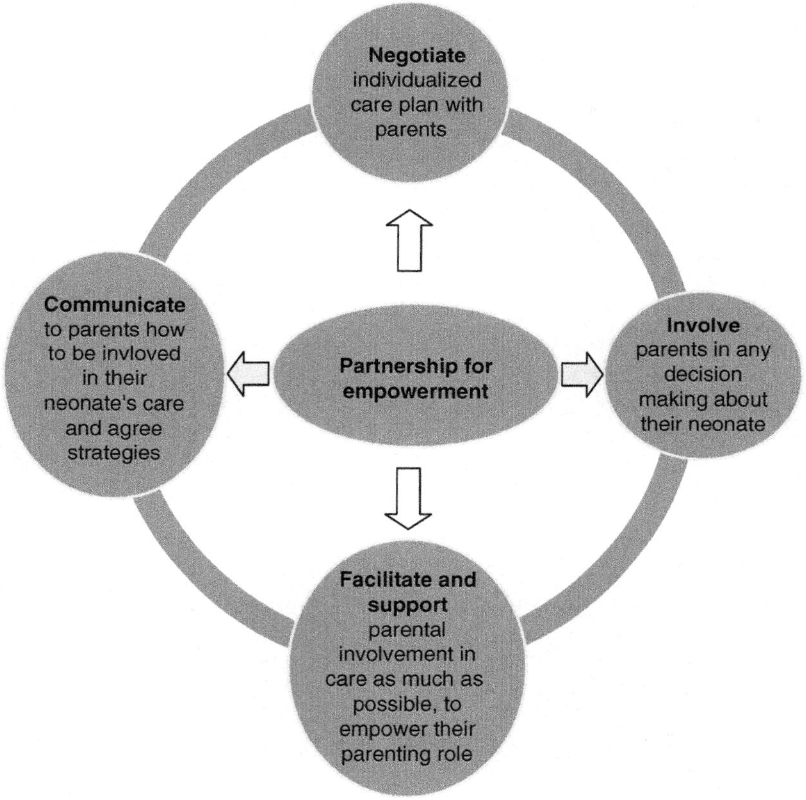

To facilitate parental involvement and enable parents to feel they have a role in their neonate's care, care should be delivered in *partnership* with them. (POPPY Steering Group, 2009; Staniszewska et al., 2012; Bracht et al., 2013).

Figure 2.31b Guide to recognizing diversity and religious/ cultural observances – DIAGRAM

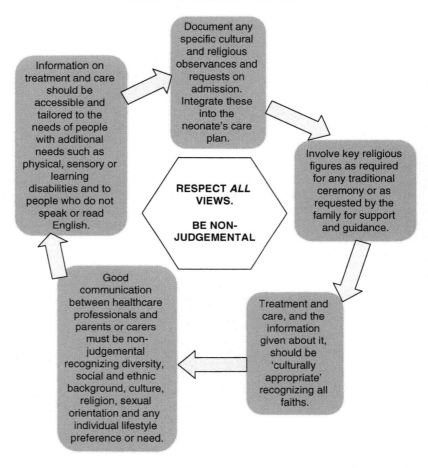

Document any specific cultural and religious observances and requests on admission. Integrate these into the neonate's care plan.

Information on treatment and care should be accessible and tailored to the needs of people with additional needs such as physical, sensory or learning disabilities and to people who do not speak or read English.

RESPECT *ALL* VIEWS.

BE NON-JUDGEMENTAL

Involve key religious figures as required for any traditional ceremony or as requested by the family for support and guidance.

Good communication between healthcare professionals and parents or carers must be non-judgemental recognizing diversity, social and ethnic background, culture, religion, sexual orientation and any individual lifestyle preference or need.

Treatment and care, and the information given about it, should be 'culturally appropriate' recognizing all faiths.

Recognizing diversity and avoiding discrimination is an essential component of the lawful care of any patient (UK DoH, 2009). Observation of the cultural elements of family and personal life is also a vital consideration (Holland and Hogg, 2010; Campinha-Bacote, 2011) and should be considered throughout a family's stay in the neonatal unit.

Ethical decision making in the neonatal unit

Psychosocial care of the family as an overarching term includes the principles of ethical decision making and palliative care. These are important areas of consideration given the complexities of current care, advances in technology and the increasing number of extremely preterm neonates surviving neonatal care. Therefore, certain care practices can involve complex and often sensitive dilemmas raising ethical debates that require clarity in order for staff and parents to make sense of such issues. Examples presented here are the issues of obtaining consent and upholding confidentiality in the neonatal unit (together as Box 2.46) followed by the delicate subject of withdrawing or withholding life-sustaining treatment in the sick and vulnerable neonate (Figure 2.31c). End of life (palliative) care then follows, to end this sub-section (Figure 2.31d).

Box 2.46   Ethical-legal issues relating to parents in the neonatal unit – CHECKLIST

Maintaining confidentiality

- Confidentiality is a legal obligation for all healthcare staff caring for neonates and their families
- Personally identifiable information with regard to neonate and family must be protected against disclosure (includes talking about patients in public places where they can be overheard, leaving any information lying around unattended and leaving computer terminals logged in, allowing open access to files)
- Access to confidential information must be on a need-to-know basis and limited to the purpose for which it is required
- Any decision to disclose information about neonate and family must be justified, in their best interest and should be documented clearly

Source: Taken from NHS England, 2014 – refer to this document for full guidance

Obtaining consent

- Consent may be obtained for clinical interventions, post-mortem examination or research participation. Where possible, all procedures should be explained
- Consent may be written, verbal or implied. For more serious, invasive procedures, consent should be a combination of verbal and written with clear documentation essential supported by a witnessed parent signature.
- Consent should be obtained by whoever is undertaking the procedure and/ or someone who is trained appropriately

(continued)

- Nurses should witness and be involved in any meeting where consent is obtained
- Documentation is a vital component of consent, particularly parental understanding and agreement of procedures
- In neonatal care, consent is obtained from someone with parental responsibility (parents if married, mother but not father if unmarried unless there is a parental responsibility agreement or the father is named on the birth certificate)
- Consent is valid only if information is understood by the parents, including why an intervention is necessary, the risks and implications
- It is good practice in neonatal care to communicate clearly from as early as possible, from neonatal admission, including provision of written information where possible (☛ see also *Communication*)
- In addition, cultural and religious factors must be considered when discussing options for interventions which may impact on parental decisions to give consent. (☛ See also Figure 2.31b)

📍 Observe any local guidance and advice along with national guidelines for any ethical-legal matters in the neonatal unit.

Source: British Association of Perinatal Medicine (BAPM)

🖐 **It is a legal and ethical requirement to gain valid consent before *any* investigation for any patient at any age. However, exceptions apply; it is not usually necessary to document consent for routine and low-risk interventions that are part of the continual and daily care of the neonate and, in emergency situations, it may not be possible to obtain parental consent in time. In this case, treatment can be given if it is deemed in the best interest of the neonate.**

Figure 2.31c Withdrawing or withholding treatment
in the neonatal unit – FLOW CHART

The decision to withdraw/withhold treatment

The decision is taken when it is deemed that continuing treatment is *not in the best interests of the neonate* and to continue treatment would cause prolonged suffering and distress. For full ethical guidance, see RCPCH (2004) and Nuffield Council (2006). Mancini et al (2014) should be referred to for full guidance in the context of palliative care.

Once a decision has been made
- Ensure both parents are present for any discussions in a private room along with any other key family members or religious figures at their request

- A time and location (e.g. hospital or home) for withdrawal of care is agreed with explanations, highlighting that the length of time to death is uncertain

⬇

- Parents should decide if they want to be present and be supported in that decision. They will also decide if they want to hold their baby or if there are any special requests to be present – e.g. clothes, toys

⬇

Physical considerations

Pain relief	Physiological monitoring	Symptom control	Fluids and nutrition	Ventilation and oxygen
Assess pain Prescribe analgesia, preferably IV route or subcutaneous/buccal/enteral as tolerated Employ non-pharmacological comfort measures ⓘ See Figure 2.33	Discontinue invasive interventions and blood tests Monitor for signs of discomfort	Assess and treat distressing symptoms appropriately	Continue in order to maintain comfort unless feeding causes pain and distress, then the decision is reviewed	Removal of ETT and cessation of ventilation support is done when fully agreed with the family

Psychosocial considerations

⬇   ⬇

Religious and spiritual care	**Psychological support**
Assess and integrate religious/spiritual needs including key religious figures and rituals as requested	Liaise with the multi-disciplinary team – e.g. psychologists, counsellors. Needs will vary. Offer appropriate choices

⬇

The goal of care is COMFORT

📍 Along with National guidance, check local policy regarding the specifics of care.

Source: Adapted with kind permission from Mancini et al. (2014). Refer to this document for full guidance in relation to palliative care following the decision to withold or withdraw treatment. This Figure can also be considered in conjunction with the BAPM (2010) guidelines for palliative care planning (See Figure 2.31d).

Figure 2.31d End-of-life (palliative) care planning in the neonatal unit – FLOW CHART

A Establishing eligibility for palliative care before or after birth		

B	**C**	**D**
Family care throughout palliative care planning and delivery Create memories Support of spiriutal, social and personal beliefs	**Communication and documentation** through the whole process Decision making Timing Primary care team(s) Key members of staff involved	**Flexible, parallel care planning** For the transition periods into and out of active, supportive and end-of-life care

E Pre-birth care antenatal, intrapartum, delivery, resuscitation decisions and planning of postnatal care

▽

F Postnatal care Supportive, comfort care, pain management, nutrition, hydration and symptom control

▽

G End-of-life care planning Location, staff involvement, preparation for changes in appearance, removal of lines and tubes, consent and parental discussions on the issues of post-mortem and organ donation

▽

H Post-death care Confirmation of death, death certification, registration of death, taking the deceased home, funeral arrangements and follow-up communication

Source: Adapted with kind permission from British Association of Perinatal Medicine (BAPM, 2010)

📍 Along with national guidance on the area of palliative care, check any local policies regarding the specifics of care.

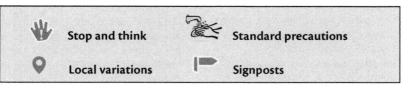

Palliative care for the neonate with a life-limiting condition is a holistic approach to care from the point of diagnosis throughout their life, death and beyond (ACT, 2009).

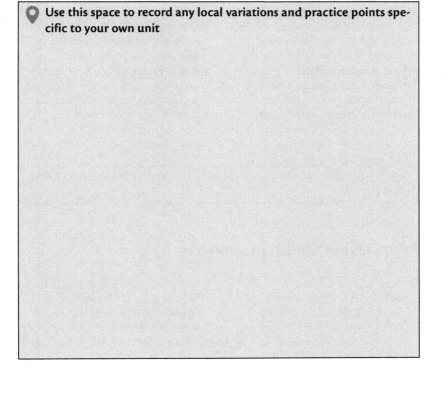

Parents and carers need to be made aware of the principles of standard precautions by explaining to them about the importance of hand hygiene and visiting policies for other family members, particularly in the winter months when viral infections are more common.

Use this space to record any local variations and practice points specific to your own unit

Parents, psychosocial care and ethical decision making: Glossary

Attachment: The nonverbal emotional relationship between a neonate and primary caregiver, defined by emotional responses to the neonates' cues, as expressed through movements, gestures and sounds (attachment behaviours).

Bonding: The intense emotional connection that the parent feels for their neonate.

Culture: The ideas, customs and social behaviour of a particular people, society or in the case of neonatal care, the family.

Empowerment: The process of increasing the capacity of individuals or groups to make choices and to transform those choices into desired actions.

Ethics: Moral principles that govern a person's behaviour or the conducting of a practice to uphold the best interests of the neonate.

Ethical decision making: The process of choosing the best alternative for achieving the best outcomes in line with individual social and moral values and the best interests of the neonate.

Family-centred care: Recognizing and valuing parents as being at the centre of the care process alongside their neonate, being responsive to parents' emotional, social and information needs and communicating clearly to support parents in how they can participate in care for their neonate.

Palliative care: Supportive care during the transition from active to end-of-life stage focusing on maintaining comfort and dignity.

Partnership: Ensuring that people have the knowledge, skills and confidence to play an active role in planning their own care; in the case of the neonatal unit, partnership with the family.

Psychosocial needs: Relates to one's psychological needs in association with the social environment.

Spiritual care: Care which recognizes and responds to the human spiritual and religious needs and beliefs when faced with ill health or trauma.

N.B. Ethical decision making and end-of-life care has a separate reference list that follows.

Parents and psychosocial care: References

BLISS – The Special Care Baby Charity (2011). *The BLISS baby charter standards.* (2nd edition) BLISS. London http://www.bliss.org.uk/improving-care/professional-development/.

Bracht, M., O'Leary, L., Lee, S., and O'Brien, K. (2013). Implementing family-integrated care in the NICU: A parent education and support program. *Advances in Neonatal Care.* 13 (2): 115–126.

Branchett, K. and Stretton, J. (2012). Neonatal palliative and end of life care: What parents want from professionals. *Journal of Neonatal Nursing.* 18 (2): 40–44.

British Association of Perinatal Medicine (2010). *Working group report. Palliative care (supportive and end of life care).* http://www.bapm.org/publications/documents/guidelines/Palliative_care_final_version_%20Aug10.pdf

Campinha-Bacote, J. (2011). Delivering patient-centered care in the midst of a cultural conflict: The role of cultural competence. *Online Journal of Issues in Nursing.* 16 (2). http://gm6.nursingworld.org/MainMenuCategories/ANAMarketplace/ANAPeriodicals/OJIN/TableofContents/Vol-16-2011/No2-May-2011/Delivering-Patient-Centered-Care-in-the-Midst-of-a-Cultural-Conflict.aspx.

Chertok, I.R.A., McCrone, S., Parker, D., and Leslie, N. (2014). Review of interventions to reduce stress among mothers of infants in the NICU. *Advances in Neonatal Care.* 14 (1): 30–37.

Feeley, N., Waitzer, E., Sherrard, K., Boisvert, L., and Zelkowitz, P. (2013). Fathers' perceptions of the barriers and facilitators to their involvement with their newborn hospitalised in the neonatal intensive care unit. *Journal of Clinical Nursing.* 22: 521–530.

Holland, K. and Hogg, C. (2010). *Cultural awareness in nursing and health care: An introductory text.* London: Hodder Arnold.

Kendall, A. and Guo, W. (2008). Evidence-based neonatal bereavement care. *Newborn and Infant Nursing Reviews.* 8 (3): 131–135.

Lee. L.A., Carter, M., Stevenson, S.B., and Harrison, H.A. (2014). Improving family centred care practices in the NICU. *Neonatal Network.* 33 (3): 125–132.

Merritt, L. (2013). Communicating with Chinese American families in the NICU using the Giger and Davidhizar transcultural model. *Neonatal Network.* 32 (5): 335–341.

Mundy, C.A. (2010). Assessment of family needs in neonatal intensive care units. *American Journal of Critical Care.* 9 (2): 156–163.

*NHS Health Scotland and Children's Hospice Association Scotland (2012). Supporting attachment in neonatal care. http://www.chas.org.uk/assets/0001/0295/Q--Early_Years____Families-Attachment-briefing_papers-Supporting_attachment_in_Neonatal_Care.pdf.

NICE. (2010). *Encouraging parental involvement in care.* http://www.nice.org.uk/guidance/qs4/chapter/quality-statement-5-encouraging-parental-involvement-in-care.

Nicholas, D.B., Hendson, L., and Reis, M D. (2014). Connection versus disconnection: Examining culturally competent care in the neonatal intensive care unit. *Social Work in Health Care.* 53 (2): 135–155.

POPPY Steering Group (2009). *Family-centred care in neonatal units; A summary of research results and recommendations from the POPPY project.* National Childbirth Trust, London. http://www.poppy-project.org.uk/resources/Poppy+report+for+PRINT.pdf.

Prior, V. and Glaser, D. (2006). *Understanding attachment and attachment disorders. Theory, evidence and practice.* London: Jessica Kingsley Publishers.

Redshaw, M.E. and Hamilton, K.E. (2010). Family centred care? Families, information and support for parents in UK neonatal units. *Arch Dis Child Fetal Neonatal edition.* 95: F365–368.

Reitmanova, S. and Gustafson, D.L. (2008). 'They can't understand it': Maternity health and care needs of immigrant Muslim women in St. John's, Newfoundland. *Maternal and Child Health Journal*. 12 (1): 101–111.

Robertson, M.J., Aldridge, A., and Curley, A.E. (2011). Provision of bereavement care in neonatal units in the United Kingdom. *Pediatric Critical Care Medicine*. 12 (3): e111.

Staniszewska, S., Brett, J., Redshaw, M., Hamilton, K., Newburn, M., Jones, N., and Taylor, L. (2012). The POPPY study: Developing a model of family-centred care for neonatal units. Worldviews on Evidence-Based Nursing. 9: 243–255.

*UK Department of Health (2009). *Religion or belief; A practical guide for the NHS*. http://www.clatterbridgecc.nhs.uk/document_uploads/EqualityandDiversity/ReligionorbeliefApracticalguide fortheNHS.pdf.

Further reading: Family care, bonding and attachment in the neonatal unit

The above documents marked * contain detailed information and can be read for further depth into both theory and practice. In addition, a sound body of theory underpins this topic and the reader may refer to the following selected open access resources to explore further.

Hopwood. R. (2010). The role of the neonatal nurse in promoting parental attachment in the NICU. *Infant*. 6 (2): 54–58. http://www.neonatalnurse.co.uk/pdf/inf_032_npp.pdf.

Obeidat, H.M., Bond, E.A., and Callister, L.C. (2009). The parental experience of having an infant in the newborn intensive care unit. *The Journal of* *Perinatal Education*. 18 (3): 23. http://www.ncbi.nlm.nih.gov/pmc/articles/PMC2730907/.

Benoit, D. (2004). Infant-parent attachment: Definition, types, antecedents, measurement and outcome. *Paediatric and Child Health*. 9 (8): 541–545. http://www.ncbi.nlm.nih.gov/pmc/articles/PMC2724160/.

Ethical decision making and end-of-life care: References

ACT. (2009). *A neonatal pathway for babies with palliative care needs*. http://www.togetherforshortlives.org.uk/assets/0000/1086/A_Neonatal_Pathway_DIAGRAM_ONLY.pdf.

British Association of Perinatal Medicine (BAPM). (2001). *Consent in neonatal clinical care*. http://www.bapm.org/publications/documents/guidelines/Staff-leaflet.pdf.

British Association of Perinatal Medicine (2010). *Working group report. Palliative care (supportive and end of life care)*. http://www.bapm.org/publications/documents/guidelines/Palliative_care_final_version_%20Aug10.pdf.

Mancini, A., Uthaya, S., Beardsley, C., Wood, D., and Modi, N. (2014). *Practical guidance for the management of palliative care on*

neonatal units (1st ed.). http://
www.chelwest.nhs.uk/services/
childrens-services/neonatal-services/
links/Practical-guidance-for-the-
management-of-palliative-care-on-
neonatal-units-Feb-2014.pdf

NHS England (2014). *Confidentiality policy.*
NHS Constitution: London. http://
www.england.nhs.uk/wp-content/
uploads/2013/06/conf-policy-1.pdf.

Nuffield Council on Bioethics (2006).
Critical care decisions in fetal and
neonatal medicine: Ethical issues.
http://nuffieldbioethics.org/
wp-content/uploads/2014/07/CCD-
web-version-22-June-07-updated.
pdf.

Royal College of Paediatrics and Child
Health (RCPCH) (2004). *Withholding*
or withdrawing life sustaining treatment
in children (2nd ed.). RCPCH: London.
http://www.gmc-uk.org/Witholding.
pdf_40818793.pdf.

Further reading: ethical decision making and end-of-life care

All the above documents contain comprehensive and detailed information on the various topics covered in this sub-section and are available as full text, open access. They should be read for further depth into both theory and practice in this topic area.

Pain management in the neonate

Neonates in hospital may experience pain because of diagnostic/thera-
peutic interventions or as a result of illness. Assessing neonates for pain is
paramount so that adequate treatment can be provided. The prevention of
pain is important not only because it is an ethical expectation of care but
also because repeated painful exposures can have deleterious consequences.
Figures 2.32 and 2.33, Box 2.47 and Tables 2.31a–c cover pain assessment and
management.

Neonatal pain assessment

A variety of neonatal pain assessment tools exist (Twycross, 2006; RCN, 2009; Cong
et al., 2013) that aim to assess physiological and behavioural responses of being
exposed to noxious stimuli. Tools can serve to aid the clinical assessment of pain
to enhance consistency between staff/carers. If a tool is used and whatever one is
chosen, there are common elements between them, summarized in Figure 2.32. In
addition, if a tool is not used then it is vital that the cues outlined here are considered. Box 2.47 lists some of the available pain assessment tools. As it is not possible
to cover all of these tools in detail, Tables 2.31a–c cover overviews of three selected
neonatal pain assessment tools, all cited within the RCN pain assessment document
(RCN, 2009). Assessment is the vital initial component in pain management which
leads onto Figure 2.33 covering an overview of strategies..

> Related topics: See also *Developmental care* and *Environmental care*
> for two areas that are closely linked with reducing stress in the neonate and
> enhancing well-being and comfort.

Figure 2.32 An overview of neonatal pain sources and cues – DIAGRAM

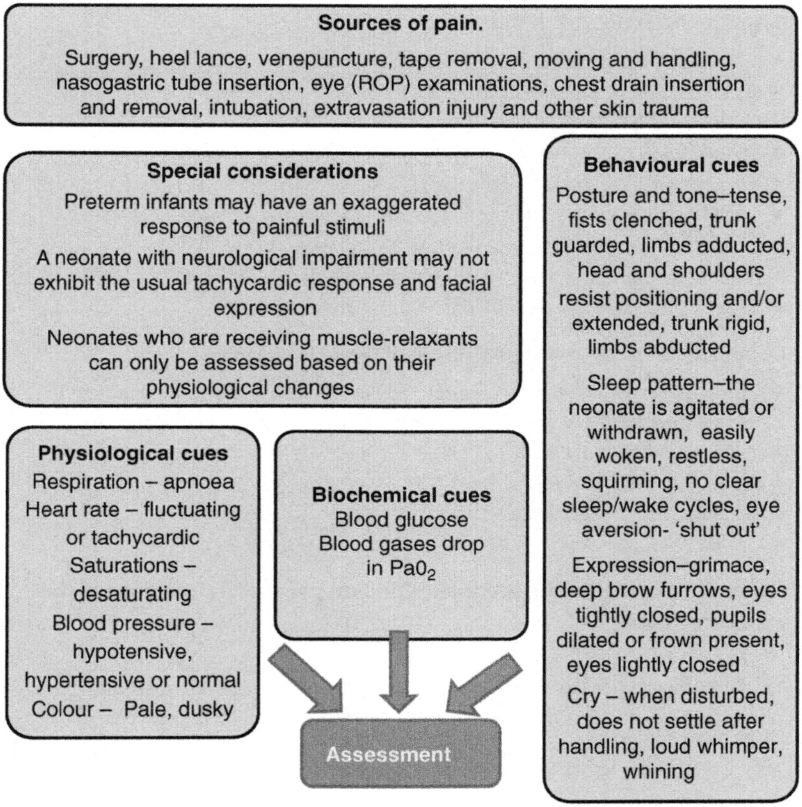

Sources of pain.

Surgery, heel lance, venepuncture, tape removal, moving and handling, nasogastric tube insertion, eye (ROP) examinations, chest drain insertion and removal, intubation, extravasation injury and other skin trauma

Special considerations

Preterm infants may have an exaggerated response to painful stimuli

A neonate with neurological impairment may not exhibit the usual tachycardic response and facial expression

Neonates who are receiving muscle-relaxants can only be assessed based on their physiological changes

Behavioural cues

Posture and tone–tense, fists clenched, trunk guarded, limbs adducted, head and shoulders resist positioning and/or extended, trunk rigid, limbs abducted

Sleep pattern–the neonate is agitated or withdrawn, easily woken, restless, squirming, no clear sleep/wake cycles, eye aversion- 'shut out'

Expression–grimace, deep brow furrows, eyes tightly closed, pupils dilated or frown present, eyes lightly closed

Cry – when disturbed, does not settle after handling, loud whimper, whining

Physiological cues

Respiration – apnoea

Heart rate – fluctuating or tachycardic

Saturations – desaturating

Blood pressure – hypotensive, hypertensive or normal

Colour – Pale, dusky

Biochemical cues

Blood glucose

Blood gases drop in PaO_2

Assessment

Assessment of pain and stress should be carried out in all neonates in any level of dependency. Signs are non-specific and not always obvious especially in very small, preterm neonates – therefore interpretation may not be straightforward. (Spence et al, 2005; Ranger et al, 2007; RCN, 2009).

Box 2.47   Pain assessment scales in neonates – CHECKLIST

Based on behavioural changes

- Neonatal Facial Coding System (NFCS)
- Infant Body Coding System (IBCS)
- Neonatal Infant Pain Scale (NIPS)
- Pain Assessment in Neonates (PAIN)
- Liverpool Infant Distress Scale (LIDS)
- Modified Behavioural Pain Scale (MBPS)
- Children's Hospital of Eastern Ontario Pain Scale (CHEOPS)
- Neonatal Assessment of Pain Inventory (NAPI)
- Wisconsin scale for preverbal/non verbal children

Combination of physiological and behavioural changes

- CRIES (acronym for crying, change in transcutaneous oxygen saturation, heart rate, blood pressure, facial expression and alteration in sleep pattern)
- Pain Assessment Tool (PAT)
- Premature Infant Pain Profile (PIPP)
- Scale for Use in Newborns (SUN)
- COMFORT Score

Generally, the higher the score obtained on pain scales, the greater the pain behaviours

Check local guidance for agreed pain assessment tool if this applies.

Selection of a pain assessment tool is dependent on individual neonatal unit choice and local guidance/preference.

Table 2.31a Neonatal pain assessment tool 1: the Wisconsin scale for preverbal/nonverbal children – SUMMARY TABLE

	0	1–2	3–4	5
Cry	No cry	Occasional whimpers	Moaning, gentle cry or whining	Consistent cry increasing in volume and duration
Facial	Calm and relaxed	Neutral expression, frowning, occasional grimace	Occasional tenseness, grimace, brow bulge, shallow nasolabial furrow	Marked distress, brow bulge, eyes squeezed shut, open mouth, deep nasal furrow
Behavioural	Moves easily, strong rhythmic suck on pacifier	Easy to console with holding, position change, winces if touched or moved	Consoles with moderate difficulty, sucks for short periods and then cries, cries if touched/moved	Inconsolable, absent suck or disorganized, high pitched cry when moved or touched
Body movement/ posture	Normal motor activity and muscle tone	Fidgeting and mild hypertonicity	Moderate agitation, intermittent flexion, moderate hypertonicity	Thrashing, flailing, consistent agitation and pronounced flexion, strong hypertonicity
Sleep	Sleeps quietly with ease of breathing, normal sleep/wake periods	Restless while asleep	Sleep periods shorter than normal, awakes easily, sleeps intermittently	Unable to sleep, sleep interrupted by jerky movements

Source: Adapted with permission from University of Wisconsin Hospital & Clinics, Madison, WI, USA; from http://prc.coh.org/pdf/Assess%20Cog%209-09.pdf

Table 2.31b Neonatal pain assessment tool 2: COMFORT scale – SUMMARY TABLE

	1	2	3	4	5
Alertness	Deeply asleep	Lightly asleep	Drowsy	Awake and alert	Awake and Hyper-alert
Calmness-Agitation	Calm	Slightly anxious	Anxious	Very anxious	Panicky
Respiratory (score only in mechanically ventilated children)	No spontaneous respiration	Spontaneous respiration	Restlessness or resistance to ventilator	Active breathing against ventilator	Fighting against the ventilator
Crying (score only in children breathing spontaneously)	Quiet breathing, no crying sounds	Occasional sobbing or moaning	Whining (monotone)	Crying	Screaming or shrieking
Physical Movement	No movement	Occasional (3 or fewer) slight movements	Frequent (more than 3) slight movements	Vigorous movements limited to extremities	Vigorous movements including torso and head
Muscle tone	Muscles totally relaxed, no muscle tone	Reduced muscle tone	Normal muscle tone	Increased muscle tone & flexion of fingers and toes	Extreme muscle rigidity & flexion of fingers and toes
Facial tension	Facial muscles totally relaxed	Normal facial tone	Tension evident in some facial muscles; not sustained	Tension evident throughout facial muscles	Facial muscles contorted and grimacing

Source: van Dijk, M, Peters, J.W, van Deventer, P and Tibboel, D. COMFORT Behavior Scale: a tool for assessing pain and sedation in infants. Am J Nurs., (2005). 105 (1), 33–6, by permission of Wolters Kluwer Health, Inc.

This tool can be used for neonates in intensive care receiving ventilation

Sum scores for all 7 indicators to gain total score

(continued)

Table 2.31b   Continued

These dimensions can also be considered as follows:					
Blood pressure (mean)	Below baseline	Normal	Infrequent elevations of >15%	Frequent elevations of >15%	Sustained elevation >15%
Heart rate	Below baseline	Normal	Infrequent elevations of >15%	Frequent elevations of >15%	Sustained elevation >15%

The original COMFORT scale comprised the following dimensions: Alertness, Calmness, Respiratory response, Movement, Mean arterial blood pressure, Heart rate, Muscle time and facial expressions

Source: Ambuel, K, Hamlett, K.W, Marx, C.M, & Blumer, J.L. Assessing Distres in Pediatric Intensive Care Environments: The COMFORT Scale, Journal of Pediatric Psychology, (1992), 17 (1), 95–109, by permission of Oxford University Press.

Table 2.31c Neonatal pain assessment tool 3: Preterm infant pain profile (PIPP) – SUMMARY TABLE

Indicator	Finding	Score
Gestational age	36 weeks and more	0
	32–35 weeks, 6 days	1
	28–31 weeks, 6 days	2
	Less than 28 weeks	3
Behavioural state	Active/awake, eyes open, facial movements	0
	Quiet/awake, eyes open, no facial movements	1
	Active/sleep, eyes closed, facial movements	2
	Quiet/sleep, eyes closed, no facial movements	3
Heart rate maximum	0–4 beats per minute increase	0
	5–14 beats per minute increase	1
	15–24 beats per minute increase	2
	25 beats per minute or more increase	3
Oxygen saturation minimum	0–2.4% decrease	0
	2.5–4.9% decrease	1
	5.0–7.4% decrease	2
	7.5% or more decrease	3

(continued)

Table 2.31c   Continued

Indicator	Finding	Score
Brow bulge	None (0–9% of the time)	0
	Minimum (10–39% of the time)	1
	Moderate (40–69% of the time)	2
	Maximum (70% of the time or more)	3
Eye squeeze	None (0–9% of the time)	0
	Minimum (10–39% of the time)	1
	Moderate (40–69% of the time)	2
	Maximum (70% of the time or more)	3
Nasolabial furrow	None (0–9% of the time)	0
	Minimum (10–39% of the time)	1
	Moderate (40–69% of the time)	2
	Maximum (70% of the time or more)	3

Sum scores for all 7 indicators to gain total score (range 0–21)

After recording the gestation, behavioural state, baseline heart rate and oxygen saturations, observe the neonate for 30 seconds following a painful event. Score physical and facial changes during this period and record

Source: Stevens, B., Johnston, C., Petryshen, P., & Taddio, A. Premature Infant Pain Profile: development and initial validation. The Clinical Journal of Pain, (1996). 12(1), 13–22, by permission of Wolters Kluwer Health, Inc.

Pain assessment should be incorporated into the neonate's care plan and should form part of holistic, regular assessment along with vital signs and other physiological cues.

Management of neonatal pain

Pain management is an essential component of neonatal care to promote optimum well-being and relieve stress in both neonate and family, both physiological and psychological. An individual approach should be used for each neonate.

Figure 2.33 Neonatal pain management – DIAGRAM

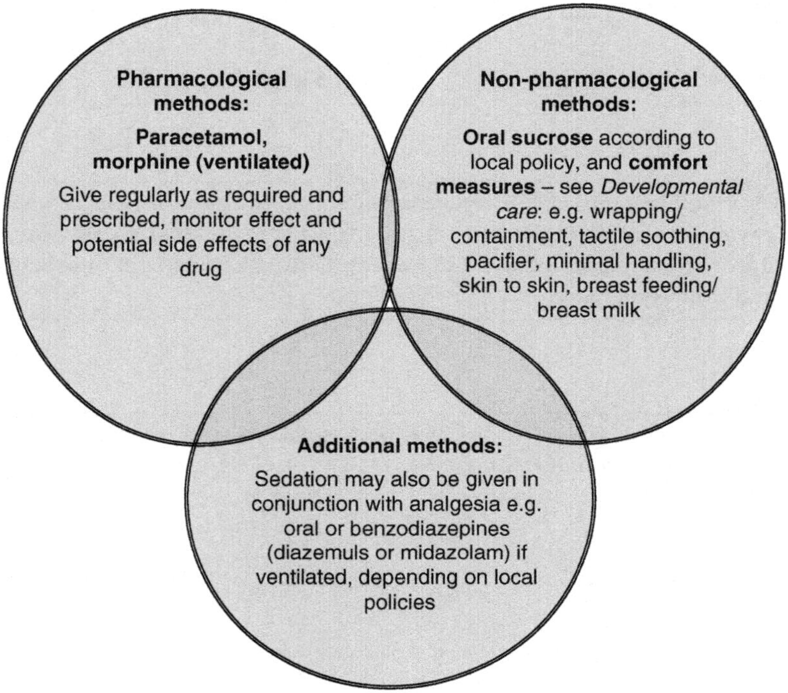

Pharmacological methods:

Paracetamol, morphine (ventilated)

Give regularly as required and prescribed, monitor effect and potential side effects of any drug

Non-pharmacological methods:

Oral sucrose according to local policy, and **comfort measures** – see *Developmental care*: e.g. wrapping/ containment, tactile soothing, pacifier, minimal handling, skin to skin, breast feeding/ breast milk

Additional methods:

Sedation may also be given in conjunction with analgesia e.g. oral or benzodiazepines (diazemuls or midazolam) if ventilated, depending on local policies

Check local guidance for agreed strategies such as the use of sucrose for procedural pain.

References: Twycross, 2006; Cooper and Petty, 2012; Meek, 2012; Shah et al., 2012; Stevens et al., 2013; Johnston et al., 2014

A combination of both approaches, pharmacological and non-pharmacological, is preferable rather than relying on just one. Use of sucrose is dependent on the individual unit and if used, there will be a policy on how, when and what to administer.

Stop and think   Standard precautions

   Local variations   Signposts

 Apply standard precautions when drawing up any analgesia or with any non-pharmacological approach to pain such as sucrose, pacifier use, use of breast milk and contact by holding. Ensure thorough hand washing and clean equipment.

 Use this space to record any local variations and practice points specific to your own unit.

Pain management: Glossary

Analgesia: Medication that acts to relieve pain.

Morphine: An analgesic and narcotic drug obtained from opium and used to relieve pain.

Pain: A highly unpleasant physical sensation caused by injury to tissues.

Paracetamol: A synthetic compound used as a drug to relieve and reduce pain and fever.

Sedation: The action of administering a sedative drug to produce a state of calm or sleep. To be distinguished from analgesia.

> The Glossaries for *Developmental care* and *Environmental care* are also relevant to this topic.

Pain management: References

Cong, X., McGrath, J., and Cusson, R. (2013). Pain assessment and measurement in neonates: An updated review. *Advances in Neonatal Care.* 13 (6): 379–395.

Cooper, S. and Petty, J. (2012). Promoting the use of sucrose as analgesia for procedural pain management in neonates: A review of the current literature. *Journal of Neonatal Nursing.* 18 (4): 121–128.

Johnston, C., Campbell-Yeo, M., Fernandes, A., Inglis, D., Streiner, D., and Zee, R. (2014). Skin-to-skin care for procedural pain in neonates. *Cochrane Database of Systematic Reviews.* Issue 1. Art. No.: CD008435.

Meek, J. (2012). Options for procedural pain in newborn infants. *Archives Disease in Childhood Education and Practice Edition.* 97: 23–28.

Ranger, M., Johnston, C.C., Anand, K.J. (2007). Current controversies regarding pain assessment in neonates. *Seminars in Perinatology.* 31 (5): 283–288.

Royal College of Nursing (RCN) (2009). *The recognition and assessment of acute pain in children clinical practice guidelines.* http://www.rcn.org.uk/__data/assets/pdf_file/0004/269185/003542.pdf.

Shah, P.S., Herbozo, C., Aliwalas, L.L., and Shah, V.S. (2012). Breastfeeding or breast milk for procedural pain in neonates. *Cochrane Database of Systematic Reviews.* Issue 12. Art. No.: CD004950.

Spence, K., Gillies, D., Harrison, D., Johnston, L., and Nagy, S. (2005). A reliable pain assessment tool for clinical assessment in the neonatal intensive care unit. *Journal of Obstetric, Gynecological & Neonatal Nursing.* 34 (1): 80–86.

Stevens, B. and Johnston, C. (1996). Premature infant pain profile: Development and initial validation. *Clinical Journal of Pain.* 12: 13–22.

Stevens, B., Yamada, J., Lee, G.Y., and Ohlsson, A. (2013). Sucrose for analgesia in newborn infants undergoing painful procedures. *Cochrane Database of Systematic Reviews.* Issue 1. Art. No.: CD001069.

Twycross, A. (2006). Managing pain during the first year of life. *Infant*. 2 (1): 10–14. http://www.infantgrapevine.co.uk/pdf/inf_007_mpd.pdf.

University of Wisconsin (2008). *Assessing pain in the nonverbal or cognitively impaired.* http://prc.coh.org/pdf/Assess%20Cog%209-09.pdf.

van Dijk, M., Peters, J.W., van Deventer, P., and Tibboel, D. (2005). The COMFORT behavior scale: A tool for assessing pain and sedation in infants. *Am J Nurs*. 105 (1): 33–36.

Further reading: neonatal pain

A sound body of theory underpins this topic and the reader may refer to the following selected open access resources to explore this further.

Henry, P.R., Haubold, K., and Dobrzykowski, T.M. (2004). Pain in the healthy full-term neonate: Efficacy and safety of interventions. *NAINR*. 4 (2). http://www.medscape.com/viewarticle/481612_2.

Slater, L., Asmerom, Y., Boskovic, D.S., Bahjri, K., Plank, M.S., Angeles, K.R., and Angeles, D.M. (2012). Procedural pain and oxidative stress in premature neonates. *The Journal of Pain*. 13 (6): 590–597. http://www.ncbi.nl+m.nih.gov/pmc/articles/PMC3367033/.

Raeside, L. (2013). Neonatal pain: Theory and concepts. *Working Papers in Health Sciences* 1: 4 Summer ISSN 2051-6266/20130020 6. http://www.southampton.ac.uk/assets/centresresearch/documents/wphs/LRNeonatal%20PainTheory%20and%20Concepts.pdf.

Quality, risk and safeguarding

This chapter focuses on a central concept in all areas of healthcare; that of quality.

Quality healthcare means doing the right thing, at the right time, in the right way, for the right person – and having the best possible results (RCN, 2011). It should be safe, effective, person-centred, timely, efficient and equitable (Institute of Medicine, 1990, cited by Health Foundation, 2014). Providing quality care also includes reducing or preventing risk and harm to the neonates in our care and ensuring we safeguard them at all times. Many of the necessary neonatal care interventions are also associated with potential iatrogenic risk to the neonate. Measures should be undertaken to avoid such harm suffered as an unfortunate consequence of care.

The integrally related areas of quality, risk and safeguarding are covered in Box 2.48, Figure 2.34, and Tables 2.32 and 2.33.

> Related topics. See also *Communication* and *Psychosocial care of the family* for links between quality care, documentation and ethical-legal issues in neonatal care.

Provision of quality care in the neonatal unit

> The principles of quality in relation to neonatal care are no different to any other area. However, we should be mindful that provision of quality, safe care *as early as possible* in a neonate's life is essential for optimum future outcomes.

Box 2.48   Quality standards in neonatal care – CHECKLIST

1. In utero and postnatal transfers for neonatal care follow network guidelines and pathways.
2. Networks, commissioners and providers of specialist neonatal care undertake an annual needs assessment and ensure each network has adequate capacity.
3. Specialist neonatal services have a sufficient, skilled and competent multi-disciplinary workforce.
4. Neonatal transfer services provide babies with safe and efficient transfers to and from specialist neonatal care.
5. Parents are encouraged and supported to be involved in planning and providing care for their neonate, and regular communication with clinical

(continued)

staff occurs throughout the care pathway. Units encourage parents to be involved in plans and processes for continuous service improvement to encourage ongoing commitment to provide family-centred care.

6. Mothers receiving specialist neonatal care are supported to start and continue breast feeding, including being supported to express milk.

7. Neonates receiving specialist neonatal care have their health and social care plans coordinated to help ensure a safe and effective transition from hospital to community care.

8. Providers of neonatal services maintain accurate data, and participate in national clinical audits and applicable research programmes. The Neonatal National Audit programme (Royal College of Paediatrics and Child Health (RCPCH), 2014) has been established aiming to inform good clinical practice in neonatal care by auditing standards.

9. Neonates receiving specialist neonatal care have their health outcomes monitored. Outcomes should be benchmarked against local and national standards BLISS (2015).

References: NICE Quality Statements (2010); BLISS (2015)

Figure 2.34 Reducing risk in the neonatal unit – FLOW CHART

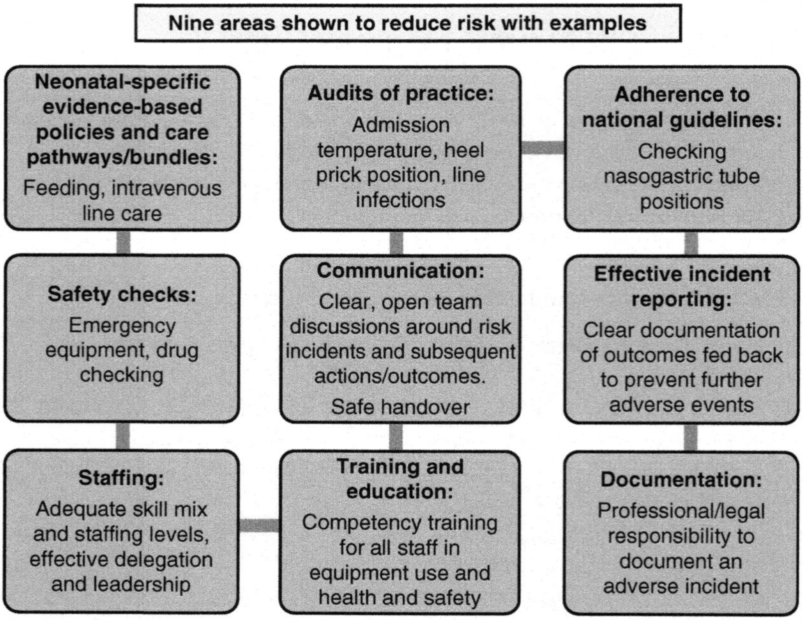

Nine areas shown to reduce risk with examples

Neonatal-specific evidence-based policies and care pathways/bundles:
Feeding, intravenous line care

Audits of practice:
Admission temperature, heel prick position, line infections

Adherence to national guidelines:
Checking nasogastric tube positions

Safety checks:
Emergency equipment, drug checking

Communication:
Clear, open team discussions around risk incidents and subsequent actions/outcomes.
Safe handover

Effective incident reporting:
Clear documentation of outcomes fed back to prevent further adverse events

Staffing:
Adequate skill mix and staffing levels, effective delegation and leadership

Training and education:
Competency training for all staff in equipment use and health and safety

Documentation:
Professional/legal responsibility to document an adverse incident

📍 Check local guidance on clinical governance strategy and incident reporting policies

References: Simpson et al. (2004) and Hamilton et al. (2007)

Local Trusts have an organization-wide strategy aimed at continuous quality improvement.

Table 2.32   Specific areas of potential iatrogenic risk in neonatal care –
SUMMARY TABLE

Area of risk	Prevention strategies
Lung damage by pressure and volume ventilation	Ventilate with minimal pressure, volume and oxygen for the least time possible
Oxygen toxicity	Resuscitate/ventilate in air unless saturations indicate a need for oxygen. Give oxygen with caution and keep to a minimum as tolerated
ETT dislodgement	Ensure careful method of securing and checking on a daily basis
Enteral tube placement	As above, secure method of fixing tube to face. Follow guidelines for passing and testing placement of enteral tubes using pH. ➧ See Box 2.34 in gastrointestinal care and feeding
IV and arterial cannula care	Hourly checks and documentation, use of Visual infusion phlebitis score (VIPS) assessment tool. ➧ See Table 2.19 in Fluid Balance and electrolytes
Umbilical catheters	As above, be aware of risks and document the perfusion of limbs. Remove any line if there is any concern with potential complication
Drug administration and errors	Reduce interruptions during drug rounds. Careful checking of drugs, in house training and neonatal staff competencies
Communication	Ensure handover is done without interruptions coupled with clear documentation each shift. Use SBAR (D) tool (situation/background/assessment/recommendation/decision). ➧ See Figure 2.14 in Communication
Infection	Follow Standard precautions and barrier nursing as applicable
Skin integrity	Careful assessment of risk to the skin. A tissue viability tool can be used. ➧ See all tools in Skin care and tissue viability sub-section

 Check local guidance and risk management policies

🖐 **Neonates, particularly those born preterm, are more prone to *iatrogenic* risk due to their vulnerability and immaturity.**

Safeguarding principles

Effective safeguarding arrangements in every area should be underpinned by two key principles. Firstly, that safeguarding is everyone's responsibility, with effective services provided by each professional and organization playing their full part; and secondly, a person(neonate)-centred approach is essential based on a clear understanding of their needs.

Table 2.33   Safeguarding principles in neonatal care – SUMMARY TABLE

Principle	What is required
The neonates' needs are paramount and put first, so that every neonate/family receives the support they need before a problem escalates	Safeguarding and planning of optimum outcomes should start from the prenatal period, through pregnancy and for the whole of the neonate's stay in the neonatal services thereafter. Cultural care should also be provided
All professionals who come into contact with neonates and families are alert to their needs and any risks of harm	Multi-disciplinary team approach Families need access to services Vulnerable groups should be targeted
All professionals share appropriate information in a timely way and can discuss any concerns about an individual case with colleagues and local authority	Interprofessional communication is a key factor in safeguarding. Identification of vulnerable families
Professionals are able to use their expert judgement to put the neonate's needs at the heart of the safeguarding system so that the right solution can be found for each individual	Staff education and training/awareness is necessary
High quality professionals contribute to whatever actions are needed to safeguard and promote a neonate's welfare	Regularly reviewing the outcomes against specific plans and outcomes is necessary – see Box 2.48 for standards and areas that can be considered

📍 Check local guidance and safeguarding policies

References: UK Government (2013)

Patient safety is paramount (Kowalski et al., 2011) and this is the core component of safeguarding (RCN, 2007, 2011; Hawdon and Hagmann, 2011).

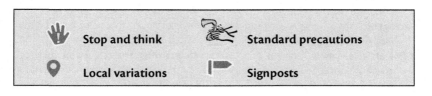

Stop and think   Standard precautions

Local variations   Signposts

The upholding of standard precautions and preventing infection is a key area known to reduce risk to the neonate.

The space below can be used to record any local variations and practice points specific to your own unit.

Quality, risk and safeguarding: Glossary

Audit: A systematic evaluation or measure resulting in an improvement in the quality of patient care.

Benchmarking: To evaluate by comparison with a standard.

Iatrogenic: Any adverse event caused by medical treatment.

Clinical Governance: A system through which NHS organizations are accountable for continuously improving the quality of their services and safeguarding high standards of care.

Quality: A distinctive attribute or characteristic. In relation to healthcare, it refers to the degree of excellence.

Risk: A probability or threat of damage, injury, liability, loss, or any other negative occurrence that is caused by external or internal factors.

Safeguarding: Protecting from harm or damage with an appropriate measure.

Standards of care: A set of guidelines for providing quality nursing care and criteria for evaluating care.

> The Royal College of Nursing (RCN, 2015) provides a detailed and comprehensive glossary on this area comprising definitions of selected terms from authoritative sources.
>
> http://www.rcn.org.uk/development/practice/clinical_governance/glossary

Quality, risk and safeguarding: References

BLISS. (2015). *National Standards.* http://www.bliss.org.uk/national-standards

Hamilton, K.E.S., Redshaw, M.E., and Tarnow-Mordi, W. (2007). Nurse staffing in relation to risk-adjusted mortality in neonatal care. *Archives of Disease in Childhood-Fetal and Neonatal Edition.* 92 (2): F99–F103.

Hawdon, J., and Hagmann, C. (2011). Support in high-risk pregnancy: Planning for specialist neonatal care. *British Journal of Midwifery.* 19 (9): 558–563.

Health Foundation (2014). What is quality? http://www.health.org.uk/about-us/what-is-quality/

Kowalski, W.J., Leef, K.H., Mackley, A., Spear, M.L., and Paul, D.A. (2011) Patient safety in the NICU: A comprehensive review. *Journal of Perinatal and Neonatal Nursing.* 25 (2): 123–132.

NICE. (2010). *Specialist neonatal care quality standards* http://publications.nice.org.uk/specialist-neonatal-care-quality-standard-qs4

RCPCH. (2014). *National Neonatal Audit Programme (NNAP).* http://www.rcpch.ac.uk/child-health/standards-care/clinical-audit-and-quality-improvement/national-neonatal-audit-programme

RCN. (2007). *Safeguarding children and young people – every nurse's responsibility. Guidance for nursing staff.* http://www.rcn.org.uk/__data/assets/pdf_file/0004/78583/004542.pdf

RCN. (2011). *Health care service standards in caring for neonates, children and young people.* https://

www.rcn.org.uk/__data/assets/
pdf_file/0010/378091/003823.pdf

RCN. (2015) *Clinical Governance:
Glossary.* http://www.rcn.org.
uk/development/practice/
clinical_governance/glossary

Simpson, J.H., Lynch, R., Grant, J.,
and Alroomi, L. (2004). Reducing

medication errors in the neonatal
intensive care unit. *Arch Dis Child Fetal
Neonatal Ed.* 89: F480–F482.

UK Government (2013). *Working
together to safeguard children: A guide
to inter-agency working to safeguard
and promote the welfare of children*
(HM Government, 2013).

Further reading: Quality, risk and safeguarding

A sound body of theory underpins this topic and the reader may refer to the
following selected open access resources to explore this further.

Health Foundation (2009). *Safety and
risk management in hospitals.* http://
patientsafety.health.org.uk/sites/
default/files/resources/safety_and_
risk_management_in_hospitals.pdf

Health Foundation (2013). *Quality
improvement made simple* (Second
edition). http://www.health.org.
uk/public/cms/75/76/313/594/
Quality%20improvement%20
made%20simple%202013.
pdf?realName=xrFN3E.pdf

Health Foundation (2014).
http://www.health.org.uk/
publications/more-than-money-
closing-the-nhs-quality-gap/?gclid=
CjwKEAjw2f2hBRCdg76qqNXfk
CsSJABYAycPcknodcRGVP3bbciq-

lSDhsdVygF7MgEN7UGvmDLzFBo
Cbpjw_wcB

NHS Commissioning Board (2013).
*Safeguarding vulnerable people in the
reformed NHS.* http://www.england.
nhs.uk/wp-content/uploads/2013/03/
safeguarding-vulnerable-people.pdf

NHS England (2013). *Neonatal critical
care.* http://www.england.nhs.uk/
wp-content/uploads/2013/06/e08-
neonatal-critical.pdf

Roland, D., Madar, J., and Connolly, G.
(2010). The newborn early warning
(NEW) system: Development of an
at-risk infant intervention system.
Infant. 6 (4): 116–120. http://
www.neonatal-nursing.co.uk/pdf/
inf_034_ris.pdf

Renal care and respiratory distress

This chapter covers the following two topics: renal assessment and respiratory distress.

Renal assessment

It is important to monitor neonatal renal function which is progressing at birth when the kidneys are still developing (Knobel and Smith, 2014). Box 2.49 covers an overview of how we monitor renal function, which includes an understanding of urinalysis, highlighting the clinical significance of various criteria.

Related topics. Attention to the renal system is closely linked to *Fluid balance and electrolytes*.

Ward-based urinalysis provides useful information on hydration levels, potential infection and tolerance to glucose (Dulczak and Kirk, 2005). It should not be overlooked when a neonate is sick in intensive care and should be used along with key laboratory testing as necessary.

Box 2.49   Renal monitoring and urinalysis – CHECKLIST

Urine collection methods
Urine bag
Cotton wool balls in nappy
Suprapubic aspiration of bladder (only if absolutely necessary)
Catheterization (rarely)

Ward-based urinalysis
Dipstick urinalysis provides information about multiple physiochemical properties of urine.

pH	The average urine is slightly acidic and usually pH is 5–6 but can vary from pH 4.8–8.5. Urine pH can be helpful in the diagnosis of renal problems/renal competency, metabolic disturbances and blood gas compensation
Specific gravity	A quick and convenient test for monitoring the concentrating and diluting power of the kidney, recognizing

(continued)

dehydration and fluid overload.

Range = 1.000 to 1.030. Low concentration (nearer 1.000) may be caused by high fluid intake. High concentration (nearer 1.030) may be caused by inadequate fluid intake/dehydration

Bilirubin   Presence of bilirubin is indicative of hepatic disease. Should be negative

Urobilinogen Normally present in urine at 0.1–1.9 mg/dl

Protein   Urine can contain a very small amount of protein (trace) but high levels can indicate infection, renal disease and immature kidneys. Should be negative or no more than a trace

Blood   Presence of blood suggests renal disease and/or infection or bleeding disorders. Should be negative

Ketones   Breakdown products of fatty acid metabolism caused by inadequate nutrition. Should be negative

Glucose   Presence of glucose is indicative of hyperglycaemia, stress, metabolic disorders or renal incompetency. Should be negative

Other laboratory urine tests:

Culture (infection screen), osmolarity (concentration), sodium (abnormal losses from kidney), metabolites (tests for metabolic disease), toxicology (tests for illicit drug use from maternal transfer to neonate)

References: Patel (2006); NICE (2007), Rogers and Saunders (2008), Falakaflaki et al. (2011)

Signs of renal failure/compromise

Plasma creatinine is the most widely used marker of renal function
Urine output should be a *minimum* of 1.0 ml/kg/hour
Weight/serum sodium and potassium/blood urea nitrogen are
also important parameters.

 Check local guidance for any specific advice on renal monitoring

References: Haycock (2003); Auron and Mhanna (2006); Knobel and Smith (2014)

	Stop and think		**Standard precautions**
	Local variations		**Signposts**

Always wear gloves and ensure thorough hand washing when handling and testing urine.

The space below can be used to record any local variations and practice points specific to your own unit.

Renal care: Glossary

Anuria: No urine output.

Glycosuria: An excess of sugar in the urine.

Ketonuria: The excretion of abnormally large amounts of ketone bodies in the urine.

Oliguria: Reduced urine output usually less than 1 ml/kg/hour in neonates.

Polyuria: Increased production of dilute urine.

Proteinuria: The presence of abnormal quantities of protein in the urine, which may indicate damage to the kidneys.

Urinalysis (dip stick): Ward-based analysis of urine to test for the presence of abnormalities.

Urine sample: Acquisition of an amount of urine to send to the laboratory for various tests such as culture and metabolites.

> The Glossary for *Fluid balance and electrolytes* is also relevant for this topic

Renal care: References

Auron, A. and Mhanna, M.J. (2006). Serum creatinine in very low birth weight infants during their first days of life. *J Perinatol.* 26 (12): 755–760.

Dulczak, S. and Kirk, J. (2005) Overview of the evaluation, diagnosis, and management of urinary tract infections in infants and children. *Urologic Nursing.* 25 (3): 185–191.

Falakaflaki, B., Mousayinasab, S.N., and Mazloomzadeh, S. (2011). Dipstick urinalysis screening of healthy neonates. *Pediatrics and Neonatology.* 52 (3): 161–164.

Haycock, G.B. (2003). Management of acute and chronic renal failure in the newborn. *Seminars Neonatology.* 8 (4): 325–334.

Knobel, R.B. and Smith, J.M. (2014). Laboratory blood tests useful in monitoring renal function in neonates. *Neonatal Network.* 33 (1): 35–40.

NICE. (2007). Urinary tract infections in children. https://www.nice.org.uk/guidance/cg54

Patel, H. (2006). The abnormal urinalysis. *Pediatric Clinics of North America.* 53 (3): 325–337.

Rogers, J. and Saunders, C. (2008). Urine collection in infants and children. *Nursing Times.* 104 (5): 40–42.

Respiratory distress

'Respiratory distress syndrome' is an actual diagnosis defined as a lack of endogenous surfactant and is the single most prevalent condition in the neonatal unit, particularly amongst the preterm population (Boyd, 2004; Pramanik and Rosenkrantz, 2012). However, term neonates can also present with it, for example, those born by lower section casearian section (LSCS) and infants born to diabetic mothers (IDM). The symptoms of respiratory distress can present with a variety of conditions as seen in the Glossary. Figure 2.35 and Box 2.50 cover a synopsis of the term 'respiratory distress' as it applies to care of the preterm neonate.

Related topics. See also *Assessment,* particularly Figure 2.3 and Tables 2.4 and 2.5, which deal with care of the preterm neonate and *Breathing* that covers ventilation strategies.

The importance of non-invasive means of respiratory support is emphasized here irrespective of the cause of the respiratory distress, i.e. to protect the lungs and prevent long-term damage (Sweet et al., 2013).

Figure 2.35 Overview of care principles for respiratory distress syndrome (RDS) – DIAGRAM

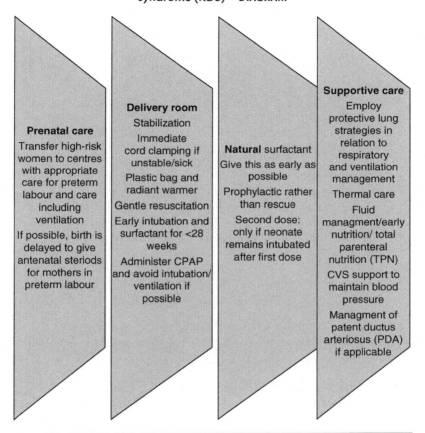

Prenatal care
Transfer high-risk women to centres with appropriate care for preterm labour and care including ventilation
If possible, birth is delayed to give antenatal steriods for mothers in preterm labour

Delivery room
Stabilization
Immediate cord clamping if unstable/sick
Plastic bag and radiant warmer
Gentle resuscitation
Early intubation and surfactant for <28 weeks
Administer CPAP and avoid intubation/ventilation if possible

Natural surfactant
Give this as early as possible
Prophylactic rather than rescue
Second dose: only if neonate remains intubated after first dose

Supportive care
Employ protective lung strategies in relation to respiratory and ventilation management
Thermal care
Fluid managment/early nutrition/ total parenteral nutrition (TPN)
CVS support to maintain blood pressure
Managment of patent ductus arteriosus (PDA) if applicable

📍 Observe local guidance on early and subsequent care of the neonate with RDS.

References: Hermansen and Lorah (2007); Stevens et al. (2007); Seger and Soll (2009); Bahadue and Soll (2012); Sweet et al. (2013)

Box 2.50   Nursing care during surfactant administration – FLOW CHART

- Preparation of surfactant – the natural preparation is kept in the refrigerator and requires warming to room temperature before use – not to be shaken
  ▽
- Endotracheal tube (ETT) tube position should be confirmed before administering surfactant to avoid erroneous instillation into one lung
  ▽
- Surfactant is administered down the endotracheal tube using a nasogastric tube (ngt) cut to a length just shorter than the ETT. Perform endotracheal suction prior to administration *only if required* and avoid afterwards for a few hours if possible
  ▽
- The neonate is laid on his or her back with the neck straight. The surfactant is given as a single bolus briefly disconnecting for a few seconds. It is important to watch for bradycardia or desaturation during administration
  ▽
- Neonates on high frequency oscillation (HFO) ventilation may be given surfactant without disconnection if suitable T-piece connectors are available
  ▽
- Following administration, lung compliance may improve quickly and ventilator requirements need to be monitored and weaned to prevent over inflation
  ▽
- Repeat dosing – following the administration of the initial dose of surfactant, the timing and necessity for further doses should be decided on an individual basis
  ▽

Non-standard use: surfactant might be used in other conditions including meconium aspiration syndrome or persistent pulmonary hypertension of the newborn (PPHN). However, the decision to use surfactant in these situations should be guided by the managing consultant on a case-by-case basis

📍 Check local guidance on surfactant administration

🖐 **When giving surfactant, watch closely for sudden changes to the neonate's oxygenation and chest expansion.**

 Stop and think   **Standard precautions**

 Local variations   **Signposts**

Always apply infection control principles to the care of any vulnerable preterm neonate with RDS who is likely to receive many invasive procedures as part of their early care and thereafter.

The space below can be used to record any local variations and practice points specific to your own unit.

Respiratory distress: Glossary

Apnoea: Interruption in breathing which may be accompanied by bradycardia.

Bronchopulmonary dysplasia (BPD): A chronic lung disorder that is most common among premature neonates who received prolonged mechanical ventilation to treat respiratory distress syndrome. BPD is defined as oxygen dependency at 36 weeks corrected age. The term is used synonymously with chronic lung disease.

Chronic lung disease: Lung damage and scarring that occurs in some neonates who are treated with oxygen and positive pressure mechanical ventilation for a prolonged period.

Meconium aspiration syndrome: A respiratory condition resulting from the fetus inhaling meconium (fetal stool) during labour and delivery following on from an episode of hypoxia.

Persistent pulmonary hypertension of the newborn (PPHN): A condition caused by a failure to convert from the fetal circulation pattern to the 'normal' pattern at birth. The pressure in the lungs therefore remains high and blood continues to be shunted from right to left through the heart ducts, causing poor oxygenation of blood to the body.

Pneumonia: A lung infection requiring treatment with antibiotics.

Pneumothorax: The presence of air in the cavity between the lungs and the chest wall (pleural cavity), causing collapse of the lung.

Protective lung strategies: Measures to limit potential lung damage during mechanical ventilation including reducing/minimizing pressure and volume as soon as possible, use of non-invasive measures such as CPAP and keeping oxygen administration to a minimum.

Pulmonary air leak: Any radiologically confirmed air leak serious enough to affect management (including pneumothorax, pulmonary interstitial emphysema, pneumopericardium, pneumoperitoneum and pneumomediastinum).

Pulmonary haemorrhage: Copious bloody secretions with clinical deterioration requiring change(s) in ventilatory management.

Respiratory distress: Characteristic signs of an inability to breathe effectively including tachypnoea, nasal flaring, grunting, chest recession and oxygen requirement.

Respiratory distress syndrome (RDS): Surfactant deficiency leading to stiff lungs with a high surface tension that are difficult to expand at birth.

Respiratory syncytial virus (RSV): RSV commonly causes viral infection in the first year of life, particularly in the winter.

Surfactant: A substance that reduces the surface tension within the lung alveoli allowing them to expand in normal breathing.

Transient tachypnoea of the newborn (TTN): A delay in the clearance of lung fluid at birth leading to a short period of mild-to-moderate respiratory compromise.

The Glossaries for *Assessment*, *Breathing* and *Oxygen therapy* are also relevant to this topic and provide further terminology.

Respiratory distress: References

Bahadue, F.L. and Soll, R. (2012). Early versus delayed selective surfactant treatment for neonatal respiratory distress syndrome. *Cochrane Database of Systematic Reviews*. Issue 11. Art. No.: CD001456. DOI: 10.1002/14651858. CD001456.pub2.

Boyd, S. (2004). Causes and treatment of neonatal respiratory distress syndrome. *Nursing Times*. 100 (30): 40–44.

Hermansen, C.L. and Lorah, K.N. (2007). Respiratory Distress in the newborn. *Am Fam Physician*. 76 (7): 987–994. http://www.aafp.org/afp/2007/1001/p987.html

Pramanik, A.K. and Rosenkrantz, T. (2012). Respiratory distress syndrome. http://emedicine.medscape.com/article/976034-overview

Seger, N. and Soll, R. (2009). Animal derived surfactant extract for treatment of respiratory distress syndrome. *Cochrane Database of Systematic Reviews*. Issue 2. Art. No.: CD007836. DOI: 10.1002/14651858.CD007836.

Stevens, T.P., Blennow, M., Myers, E.H., and Soll, R. (2007). Early surfactant administration with brief ventilation vs. selective surfactant and continued mechanical ventilation for preterm infants with or at risk for respiratory distress syndrome. *Cochrane Database of Systematic Reviews*. Issue 4. Art. No.: CD003063.

Sweet, D., Bevilacqua, G., Carnielli, V., Greisen, G., Plavka, R., Saugstad, O., Simeoni, U., Speer, C.P., VallsiSoler, A., and Halliday, H. (2013). European consensus guidelines on the management of neonatal respiratory distress syndrome – 2013 Update. *Neonatology*. 103: 353–368. DOI: 10.1159/000349928

Skin care and surgical nursing practice

This chapter covers the following two topics: Skin care and care issues relating to the surgical neonate.

Skin care and tissue viability

The skin of a newborn, particularly if born preterm, has a relatively poor barrier function with a greater risk of injury from pressure and shearing forces than older infants and children (Irving, 2006; Blume-Peytavi et al., 2014). This can increase the risk of infection, discomfort, excoriation or epidermal stripping, particularly if the skin is immature or oedematous because of illness. Skin care can therefore be challenging. The important practice points for skin care in relation to general skin assessment, tissue viability, risk assessment, prevention/management of pressure sores and wound management as a whole are outlined in Boxes 2.51a–b, Tables 2.34a–d and Figures 2.36a–b

> Related topics. See also *Assessment* to see how skin assessment is part of the holistic approach and *Hygiene needs* in the neonate.

Box 2.51a   Neonatal skin assessment – CHECKLIST

- Check for skin integrity at birth and then regularly thereafter in line with timing of care procedures. ▶ See also *Hygiene*. Observe colour, appearance, level of moisture/dryness and if the skin is intact.
- Observe for specific *risks*: skin oedema, poor skin perfusion, muscle relaxants and gestational age; the preterm neonate has immature and more fragile skin. ▶ See Tables 2.34a (i) and (ii)
- Pay attention to vulnerable sites; e.g. nappy and umbilical area, lines, tubes and/or adhesives (nasal CPAP, ETT (lips), gastric tubes), probe sites (e.g. saturation, transcutaneous), IV and arterial line sites. During immobility, observe pressure sites: common vulnerable areas being the occiput, heels and the back of the ears. ▶ See Figure 2.36a and Table 2.34c.
- Observe for areas of trauma and increased skin vulnerability: epidermal stripping, tearing from adhesive and friction, contact injury (chemicals, moisture, irritants) such as nappy dermatitis and ischaemic injury
- Assess and follow specific instructions according to risk and/or from specialist Tissue Viability Nurse (TVN) in the presence of surgical wounds. ▶ See Table 2.34d

(continued)

🦫 Standard precautions should be applied to any skin assessment and care particularly if there is any excoriation or concern about skin integrity.

📍 Check local guidance on skin assessment

References: Baharestani (2007); Baharestani and Ratliff (2007) Hughes (2011); Jones (2013); August et al (2014).

🖐 **Presence of vernix, lanugo hair (<34 weeks gestation), xerosis (in post-term) and harmless rashes (e.g. milia, erythema toxicum) are normal findings.**

Table 2.34a(i)   Assessing tissue viability risk 1 – SUMMARY TABLE

Skin viability assessment tool 1

Intensity/duration of pressure			
Score	**3**	**2**	**1**	**0**
Physical condition	Gestation <28 weeks	28–32 weeks	>33–<38 weeks	>38 weeks
Mobility	Immobile	Very limited	Slightly limited	No limitations
Activity	No activity	Very limited	Slightly limited	No limitations
Sensory perception	Completely limited	Very limited	Slightly limited	No impairment
Skin tolerance and structure			
Moisture	Constantly moist	Very moist	Occasionally moist	Rarely moist
Friction	Significant problem	Problem	Potential problem	No problem
Nutrition	Very poor	Inadequate	Adequate	Excellent
Tissue perfusion and oxygenation	Extremely compromised	Compromised	Adequate	Excellent

(continued)

Table 2.34a(i)   Continued

Scores

0–5: Low risk, 6–10: At risk, 11–19: High risk, >20: Very high risk

Plan care accordingly – see Table 2.34b

 Check local guidance on skin assessment

Source: Adapted from Ashworth C., Briggs L., Design and implementation of a neonatal Tissue Viability Assessment Tool on the newborn intensive care unit. Infant. 7 (6). Pages 191–94. (2011), with permission from Infant journal and tool author, Louise Briggs with thanks.

Table 2.34a(ii)   Assessing tissue viability risk 2 – SUMMARY TABLE

Skin viability assessment tool 2

Risk factor	Score
Neonate cannot be moved or deterioration in condition/under general anaesthetic >2 hours	20
Unable to change position without assistance/cannot control body movement	15
Some mobility	10
Normal mobility for age	0
Equipment/objects/hard surfaces pressing or rubbing on skin	15
Significant anaemia	1
Persistent pyrexia	1
Poor peripheral perfusion (cold extremities/capillary refill >2–3 seconds/cool mottled skin)	1
Inadequate nutrition	2
Low serum albumin	1

Scores

0: No risk, >10: At risk, >15: High risk >20: Very high risk
Plan care accordingly – see Table 2.34b

 Check local guidance on skin assessment

Source: Tool reproduced with kind permission from author Jane Willock and adapted version from Health Improvement Scotland. Willock, J, Baharestani, MM and Anthony D. (2007). The development of the Glamorgan paediatric pressure ulcer risk assessment scale. Journal of Children's and Young People's Nursing. Copyright © [2007]. MA Healthcare Ltd. Reproduced by permission of MA Healthcare Ltd.

Regular skin assessment including any areas of concern, risk or actual skin damage must be incorporated into a neonate's care plan.

Table 2.34b   Nursing actions according to tissue viability risk –
SUMMARY TABLE

Category	Suggested action
Not at risk/ low risk	Continue to reassess daily and every time condition changes
At risk	Inspect skin with all care procedures. Relieve pressure by regular position changes. Re-site probes more frequently, use of protective dressing for cannulas and endotracheal tubes, loosen tapes, regular checks of areas.
High risk	Inspect skin with each repositioning/cares as above. Use of adjuncts to relieve pressure e.g. gel mattress. Seek advice from TVN.
Very high risk	Inspect skin at least hourly if condition allows. More regular probe changes. Avoid adhesive tapes. Refer to TVN.

Ensure Standard precautions are maintained with any skin assessment and care particularly when there are concerns about skin viability.

Check local guidance on choice of skin viability risk assessment tool, recommended actions and subsequent care planning.

For all risk categories, skin assessment should be clearly documented and handed over from shift to shift.

Figure 2.36a Prevention and management of pressure ulcers in the neonate – FLOW CHART

Assessment of skin and risk of pressure ulcers

- Perform skin assessment – see Box 2.51a
- Perform risk assessment – use a tool validated and adapted for this population such as the Braden Q or Glamorgan scale. SeeTables 2.34a (i) and (ii)
- Use tools to support clinical judgement
- Document findings

Prevention

- Regular and documented skin assessment – see above
- Take particular note of skin changes in the occipital area, ears and heels
- Note skin temperature and any blanching, erythema or skin discolouration
- Reposition neonate every 4 hours or more frequently if required
- Relieve pressure on the scalp/head, heels, ears and knees if prone
- Use a foam cot mattress or overlay for at-risk neonates
- Consider a pressure redistributing device/pillow for neonates at risk of occipital pressure ulcers
- All above should be part of an individualised care plan

Management

- Document the surface area and depth of any pressure ulcer
- Categorize any pressure ulcer using the NPUAP-EPUAP (2009) classification system (grades 1 to 4) – see Table 2.34c
- Assess fluid balance and ensure hydration is optimized
- Consider using specialist support devices (see above)
- Use dressings that promote a warm, moist healing environment to treat grade 2, 3 and 4 pressure ulcers – see Box 2.51b and Figure 2.36b
- Debridement (autolytic) may be necessary with a chosen dressing – seek advice from Tissue Viability Nurse (TVN)
- Antibiotics may be required for infected pressure ulcers

 Standard precautions should be applied to any pressure ulcer care

🔘 Check local guidance on assessment and care of pressure ulcers in the neonatal unit

References: EPUAP/NPUAP (2009); *Reference:* NICE Guideline 179 (2014). http://www.nice.org.uk/guidance/cg179

Table 2.34c   Pressure ulcer classification system – SUMMARY TABLE

Category/Stage I: non-blanchable erythema	Intact skin with non-blanchable redness of a localized area usually over a bony prominence
Category/Stage II: partial thickness	Partial thickness loss of dermis presenting as a shallow open ulcer with a red pink wound bed, without slough. May also present as an intact or open/ruptured serum-filled or sero-sanginous filled blister. Presents as a shiny or dry shallow ulcer without slough or bruising
Category/Stage III: Full thickness skin loss	Full thickness tissue loss. Subcutaneous fat may be visible but bone, tendon or muscle is *not* exposed. Slough may be present but does not obscure the depth of tissue loss
Category/Stage IV: Full thickness tissue loss	Full thickness tissue loss with exposed bone, tendon or muscle. Slough or scarring may be present

Source: Reprinted with permission from: European Pressure Ulcer Advisory Panel and National Pressure Ulcer Advisory Panel. Prevention and treatment of pressure ulcers: quick reference guide. Washington DC: National Pressure Ulcer Advisory Panel; 2009. http://www.npuap.org/wp-content/uploads/2012/02/Final_Quick_Prevention_for_web_2010.pdf

✋ Neonates considered to be 'at risk' of pressure ulcers are identified after assessment using clinical judgment and/or an agreed risk assessment tool (NICE, 2014). 'High risk' factors include limited mobility, immaturity, nutritional deficiency, previous or existing areas of skin breakdown and numerous invasive IV sites or tubes.

Table 2.34d   Neonatal wound assessment – SUMMARY TABLE

Classification of wound can be undertaken by observing the colour which indicates the stage of wound healing and/or any presence of infection	
Wound colour Pink: New growth of skin Red: Granulating, new vascular connective tissue Yellow: slough (dead cells) Green/yellow: Infected Black: Necrotic tissue	
Wound site	Document site(s) and indicate on care plan where the wound is.
Wound size	Width, breadth and depth-record all. Provide possible drawing in the care plan of shape and size of wound.

(continued)

Table 2.34d Continued	
Thickness/ depth	Partial thickness- damaged epidermis and dermis. Full thickness- also involves subcutaneous tissue and below.
Exudate	Serous fluid, blood or pus.
Odour	None to mild to obvious.
Skin integrity	Surrounding skin-assess colour, moisture, breakdown, oedema, pain, rash, skin changes, infection
Skin maturity	Gestation- observe presence of translucency, friability and integrity which indicates preterm skin.
Pain	Present all the time or at dressing change only

○ Check local guidance on wound assessment

References: Taquino (2000); Clifton-Koeppel (2006); Baharestani (2007).

A systematic assessment of any wound is vital as this provides baseline information on which to assess healing and effectiveness of management given.

Box 2.51b   Neonatal wound care principles – CHECKLIST

- Causes of wounds in the neonate: trauma (epidermal stripping, tearing), surgical incisions, contact excoriation (chemicals, moisture, urine/stool), extravasation, thermal injury, pressure ulcers, ischaemia and congenital (epidermolyis bullosa, gastroschisis, myelomeningocele).
- Protect any wound from trauma with non-adherent dressing/covering.
- Deeper, more significant wounds that are granulating heal better with moist wound healing and a dressing that promotes this. This enhances the optimum environment for epithelialization, growth of new skin tissue and the prevention of trauma from the wound drying out.
- Use a dressing that maintains an ideal environment for wound healing (low adherent, vapour permeable). Dressing choice will depend on type and depth of wound and level of exudate- see Figure 2.36b.
- Superficial wounds (e.g. skin excoriation) can be exposed to air.
- Wound cleansing may be necessary in the presence of debris, bacteria or necrosis. Routine cleansing of all wounds, however is not necessary.

(continued)

▮ᐳ   See also guidelines for extravasation injuries and stoma care – see *Fluid balance and electrolytes* and *Surgical nursing practices*

Standard precautions should be applied to any wound care practice to prevent infection which can complicate the healing process.

◉ Check local guidance on wound care

References: Taquino (2000); Irving (2006); Irving et al. (2006)

Whatever the cause, the aims of wound care are the same: to protect the wound area, to promote optimum healing and resumed skin integrity, to prevent breakdown and if necessary, to provide gentle cleansing and treatment in the presence of infection.

Figure 2.36b Wound care overview – FLOW CHART

| Wound identified |

▽   ▽

| Wound caused by planned event (surgery, cannulation, puncture) Is it clean and dry? **No action required** | Wound caused by iatrogenic event or excessive pressure/unexpected occurrence? Or wound breaking down/discharge present? **Continue below** |

▽

| Refer and seek advice from Tissue Viability Nurse (TVN) |

▽

| Assess wound using Table 2.34d |

▽

| Apply wound care principles – ☐ See Box 2.51b |

| Carry out wound care according to classification – see below |

Classification	Aim of care	Suggested dressing(s)
1. Pink (epithelializing)	Keep wound moist/warm and protect	Hydrocolloid sheets are self-adhesive, absorb fluid and are impermeable to bacteria and/or soft, non-adherent silicone layer
2. Red (granulating)	Keep wound moist/warm, protect, promote granulation and manage exudate	Amorphous hydrogel with semi-permeable non-occlusive dressing
3. Yellow (sloughy)	Debridement and management of exudate	As for 1 and 2 above
4. Green (infected)	Prevent any further infection	Hydrocolloid fibrous dressing with foam
5. Black (necrotic)	Debridement and management of exudate	As for 1 and 2 above

▽

| Devise plan of care and frequency of dressing change with TVN and document. Review wound appearance and care with each dressing change until healing has been achieved |

🪶 Remember standard precautions when dealing with any type of wound and dressing.

🔵 Check local guidance on wound care and dressings

Reference: South Central Neonatal Network Quality Care Group (2012)

Management of an individual wound will be determined by how that wound is classified as seen above.

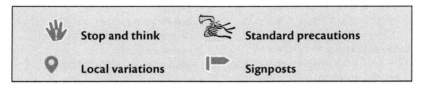

Stop and think   Standard precautions

Local variations   Signposts

Vigilant infection control precautions must be applied with any wound management. Wash hands before and after any procedure and wear gloves/aprons according to local guidelines.

Use this space to record any local variations and practice points specific to your own unit.

Skin care: Glossary

Epidermal stripping: Removal of one or more layers of the stratum corneum (outer layer of the epidermis) of the skin following removal of adhesive tape or dressings.

Epithelialization: The process of becoming covered with epithelium, an important process in the proliferation phase of skin healing, following the inflammation stage and leading to the final remodeling stage.

Erythema: Redness of the skin.

Excoriation: Abrasion of the skin where it may be torn and damaged.

Granulation: Part of the skin healing process in which new connective tissue and capillaries forms around the edges of a wound, part of the final remodeling stage.

Keratin: Fibrous structural protein of epithelial cells in the stratum corneum of the skin.

Pressure area: An area of the body prone to injury from pressure at rest.

Pressure sore: An area of skin breakdown caused by prolonged pressure and/or immobility.

Slough: A layer of dead tissue separated from the underlying or surrounding living tissue, as in a wound.

Stratum corneum: The outermost layer of the skin's epidermis acting as a mechanical barrier.

Vernix: Waxy white substance on newborn skin.

Xerosis: Skin dryness.

Skin care: References

Ashworth, C. and Briggs, L. (2011). Design and implementation of a neonatal tissue viability assessment tool on the newborn intensive care unit. Infant. 7 (6): 191–194. http://www.neonatal-nursing.co.uk/pdf/inf_042_lem.pdf

August, D.L., Edmonds, L., Brown, D.K., Murphy, M., and Kandasamy, Y. (2014). Pressure injuries to the skin in a neonatal unit: Fact or fiction. *Journal of Neonatal Nursing.* 20 (3): 129–137.

Baharestani, M.M. and Ratliff, C.R. (2007). The national pressure ulcer advisory panel. Pressure sores in neonates and children. An NPUAP white paper. *Advanced Skin Wound Care.* 20 (4): 208–220.

Baharestani, M.M. (2007). An overview of pediatric and neonatal wound care knowledge and considerations. *Ostomy Wound Management.* 53 (6): 34–36, 38, 40.

Blume-Peytavi, U., Hauser, M., Stamatas, G.N., Pathirana, D., and Garcia Bartels, N. (2012). Skin care practices for newborns and infants: Review of the clinical evidence for best practices. *Pediatric Dermatology.* 29: 1–14.

Clifton-Koeppel, R. (2006). Wound care after peripheral intravenous extravasation: What is the evidence? *Newborn and Infant Nursing reviews.* 6 (4): 202–212.

European Pressure Ulcer Advisory panel (EPUAP) and National Pressure Ulcer Advisory Panel (NPUAP) (2009). *Pressure ulcer prevention: Quick reference guide.* http://www.npuap.org/wp-content/uploads/2012/02/

Final_Quick_Prevention_for_web_2010.pdf

HealthCare Improvement Scotland (HIS) (2009). *Paediatric risk assessment tool.* http://www.healthcareimprovement scotland.org/our_work/patient_safety/tissue_viability_resources/paediatric_glamorgan_tool.aspx

Hughes, K. (2011). Neonatal skin care: Advocating good practice in skin protection. *British Journal of Midwifery.* 19 (12): 773–775.

Irving, V. (2006). Wound care for preterm neonates. *Infant.* 2 (3): 102–106.

Irving, V., Bethell, E., and Burton, F. (2006). Neonatal wound care; Minimising trauma and pain. *Wounds UK.* 2 (1): 33–41.

Jones, K. (2013). Advice to promote healthy neonatal skin and treat common skin disorders. *British Journal of Midwifery.* 21 (4): 244–247.

NICE. (2014). *Pressure ulcers: Prevention and management of pressure ulcers.* http://www.nice.org.uk/guidance/cg179

South Central Neonatal Network Quality Care Group (2012). *Guideline framework for neonatal wound care.* http://www.networks.nhs.uk/nhs-networks/thames-valley-wessex-neonatal-network/documents/guidelines/Wound%20Guideline.pdf/at_download/file.

Taquino, L.T. (2000). Promoting wound healing in the neonatal setting: Process versus protocol. *Journal of Perinatal and Neonatal Nursing.* 14 (1): 104–118.

Willock, J, Baharestani, MM and Anthony D. (2007). The development of the Glamorgan paediatric pressure ulcer risk assessment scale. *Journal of Children's and Young People's Nursing.* 1 (5): DOI: http://dx.doi.org/10.12968/jcyn.2007.1.5.27446

Further reading: Skin care and hygiene

A sound body of theory underpins this topic and the reader may refer to the following selected open access resources to explore this further.

Baharestani, M.M. (2007). An overview of neonatal and pediatric wound care knowledge and considerations. *Ostomy Wound Management.* 53 (6): 34–55. http://www.o-wm.com/content/an-overview-neonatal-and-pediatric-wound-care-knowledge-and-considerations

Crozier, K. and Macdonald, S. (2010). Effective skin-care regimes for term newborn infants: A structured literature review. *Evidence Based Midwifery.* 11 September 2010 https://www.rcm.org.uk/content/effective-skin-care-regimes-for-term-newborn-infants-a-structured-literature-review

Darmstadt, G.L. and Dinulis, D.G. (2000). Neonatal skin care. *Pediatric Clinics of North America.* 47 (4): 757–782. http://www.pediatric.theclinics.com/article/S0031-3955(05)70239-X/abstract

Surgical nursing practice

Knowledge of the nursing care practices relating to the surgical neonate is a substantial topic and to go through each surgical condition, particularly the whole repertoire of congenital structural anomalies (see Glossary) is beyond the scope of this book. However, some common practices can apply more broadly to any surgical case, which is the focus of the current unit. Boxes 2.52 and 2.53 and Figures 2.37–2.39 address some individual care topics and practices that anyone working with a surgical neonate would find useful; namely, pre- and post-operative checklist, gastric decompression, replogle tube care, stoma care and fluid/feeding issues.

> Related topics. See also *Gastrointestinal care and feeding* which contains further detail on Necrotizing Enterocolitis (NEC) and recognizing GIT obstruction. The section on *Vomiting* is also relevant.

> **Optimum preparation both prior to surgery and in the post-operative period aims to ensure that the neonate is safe, physiologically ready to cope with anaesthesia and surgery and that the family is psychologically prepared (Dickson and Smith, 2006).**

Box 2.52   Pre- and post-operative care of the surgical neonate – CHECKLIST

Pre-operative checklist
The following should be completed and documented (RCN, 2011):

- Patient details and assessment overview. Consider the systems (see *Assessment*)
- Baseline observations including temperature
- Blood results as applicable (full blood count, clotting)
- Assessment of pain
- Record of any previous events in surgery
- Pre-operative fasting information (when NBM started)
- Pre-operative safety checklist
- Discussion with parents
- Consent form signed following clear discussion
- Risk assessment to ensure transfer to and from theatre – see below

Specific conditions: some examples
- Acute intestinal obstruction including NEC – gastric decompression (NGT in place), observe for perforation (de la Hunt, 2006; Kelly et al., 2008)
- **Signs of intestinal obstruction-abdominal distension, bilious vomiting, absent bowel sounds, failure to pass meconium or stool.** See *Gastrointestinal care and feeding and* Box 2.35

(continued)

- Oesophageal atresia – replogle tube drainage (Johnson, 2005; Holland et al., 2010)
- Gastroschisis – cling film wrap/protection of exposed gut (Lund and Berrios, 2007)
- Congenital diaphragmatic hernia – stabilization prior to theatre (Leeuwen and Fitzgerald, 2014)

Post-operative checklist

The following should be completed and documented:

- As above, ensure safe transfer back to unit by risk assessment
- Recovery assessment details following procedure and anaesthetic
- Post-operative observations – ascertain frequency
- Respiratory management post-operatively and oxygen requirement
- Prescription chart with appropriate analgesia/nurse-controlled analgesia/ assess pain
- Fluid/feeding management (varies depending on neonate and condition plus how much bowel is compromised) (Brasher et al., 2014)
- Wound care plan – see *Skin Care* section Table 2.34d, Box 2.51b and Figure 2.36b
- Summary of operation, signed/dated by surgeon with clear post-operative instructions including any potential risks (blood loss, significant changes to vital signs)
- Explanations to parents

Specific conditions

Follow post-operative instructions for individual conditions, for example:

- Resection for acute intestinal obstruction including NEC – continue gastric decompression, and if applicable, stoma assessment
- Oesophageal atresia – ensure trans-anastomotic tube (nasogastric tube that passes the surgical oesophageal wound) is not dislodged
- Gastroschisis – care of the silo sac over the exposed abdominal contents
- Congenital diaphragmatic hernia – ventilation management is continued until pulmonary hypertension is resolved

Risk assessment for transfer to and from theatre

Low risk: No oxygen therapy, good oxygen saturations in air, alert and clinically stable

Medium risk: Oxygen requirement and signs of respiratory distress

High risk: Oxygen therapy >40%, requiring ventilation support

Assessment of risk will determine who may be required to accompany neonate for transfer and equipment needed: transfer bag, suction, oxygen cylinder

Standard precautions should be applied to pre- and post-operative practices to prevent any infection to the neonate during and after the whole surgical experience.

Check local guidance on pre- and post-operative care

For full assessment criteria see link to RCN, (2011)

Gastric decompression

One of the most important, and yet simple procedures to undergo in the surgical neonate is insertion of a short, wide-bore gastric tube for free drainage, gastric decompression and prevention of abdominal perforation. This is vital for any neonate with abdominal distension or suspected obstruction from whatever cause.

Figure 2.37 Gastric decompression – FLOW CHART

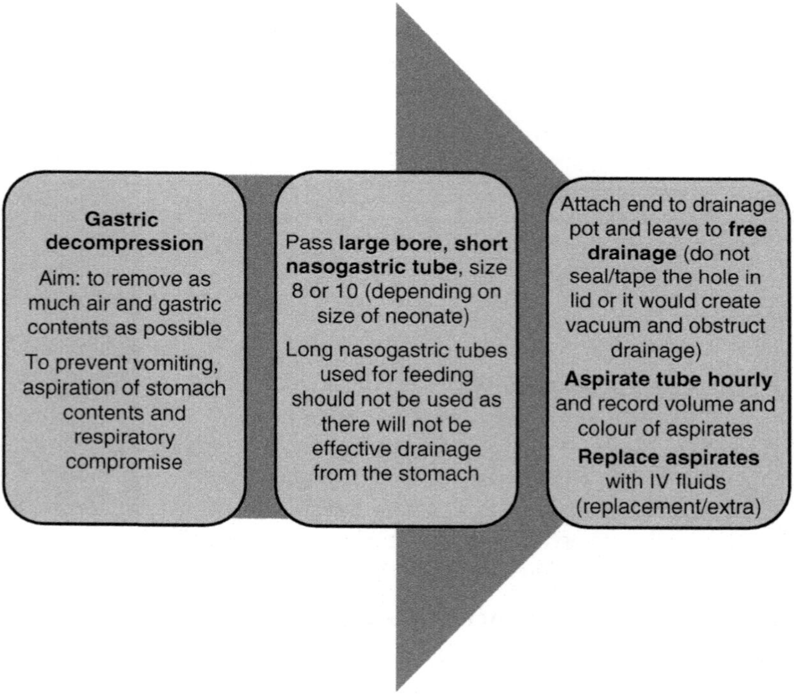

Gastric decompression	**Pass large bore, short nasogastric tube**, size 8 or 10 (depending on size of neonate)	Attach end to drainage pot and leave to **free drainage** (do not seal/tape the hole in lid or it would create vacuum and obstruct drainage)
Aim: to remove as much air and gastric contents as possible	Long nasogastric tubes used for feeding should not be used as there will not be effective drainage from the stomach	**Aspirate tube hourly** and record volume and colour of aspirates
To prevent vomiting, aspiration of stomach contents and respiratory compromise		**Replace aspirates** with IV fluids (replacement/extra)

Remember standard precautions when handling any body fluid such as gastric aspirate- wear gloves, perform careful hand washing and follow local guidelines for disposal.

Check local guidance for gastric decompression practice.

For *any* suspicion of acute intestinal obstruction from any cause, it is absolutely essential to remove the feeding tube and immediately insert a short, wide bore nasogastric tube on full drainage.

Replogle tube care

A replogle tube is a double lumen tube used to remove secretions from the upper gastrointestinal tract and prevent aspiration (Johnson, 2005; Holland et al., 2010). It is most commonly used for oesophageal atresia when the tube is passed into the oesophageal pouch (blind end) to clear secretions.

Figure 2.38 Replogle tube care – FLOW CHART

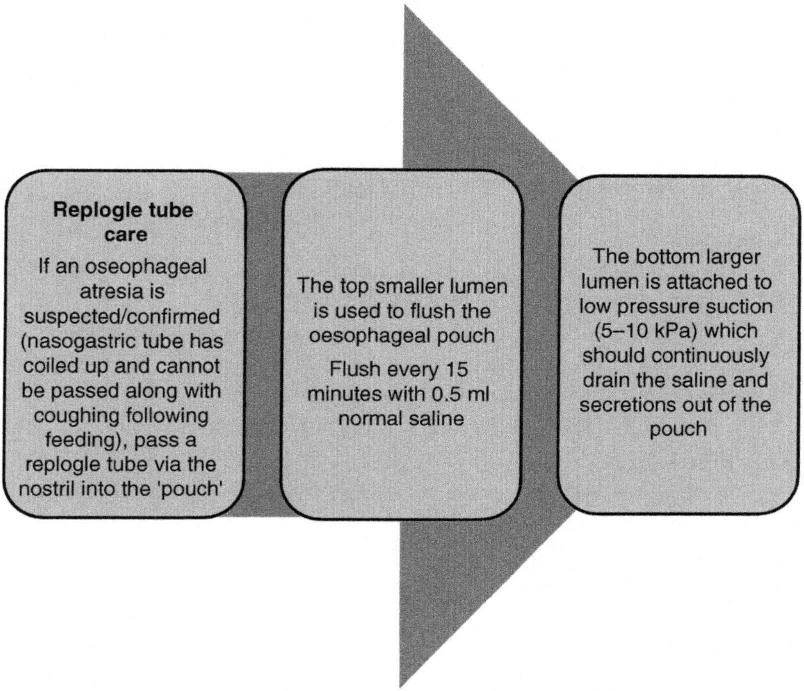

Replogle tube care

If an oseophageal atresia is suspected/confirmed (nasogastric tube has coiled up and cannot be passed along with coughing following feeding), pass a replogle tube via the nostril into the 'pouch'

The top smaller lumen is used to flush the oesophageal pouch

Flush every 15 minutes with 0.5 ml normal saline

The bottom larger lumen is attached to low pressure suction (5–10 kPa) which should continuously drain the saline and secretions out of the pouch

Remember standard precautions when handling any tube inserted into the gastrointestinal tract

Check local guidance for replogle tube care.

Continuous suction is necessary to ensure adequate clearance of secretions from the upper gastrointestinal tract and prevent them from entering the lungs.

Stoma care

A stoma may be formed following resection of any part of the small or large bowel when a primary anastomosis is not possible. The bowel is therefore brought out to the surface of the abdomen either as a loop or as two ends comprising a proximal, functioning stoma (top of the bowel which eliminates stool) and a distal 'mucous fistula' (which leads to the lower part of bowel and to the anus).

> Observation of both the stoma and the surrounding skin is an essential part of post-operative assessment (Rogers, 2003; Harrell-Bean and Klell, 2006).

Box 2.53   Neonatal stoma care – CHECKLIST

Assessment
- Colour of stoma (should be deep red/pink)
- Position of stoma (should be slightly raised)
- Report/refer if: the stoma bleeds excessively, prolapses out or retracts in, turns dark or bluish in colour and/or if the stoma losses become increasingly watery
- Observe the skin for signs of excoriation/rashes/epidermal stripping

Care principles
- Routine stoma care includes: emptying of stoma bag of stool/flatus, change of stoma bag, care of peristomal skin

Stoma and stoma bag care
- Cover stoma initially with a paraffin gauze dressing then add a dry gauze layer over this
- When the stoma becomes active, a stoma bag should be fitted
- Ensure the flange of the bag is cut and fits closely around the stoma site with minimum skin exposed to stool and stoma losses which can cause excoriation. ▶ See *Skin care*
- Skin protective agents may be used on advice of the stoma specialist if skin starts to become excoriated.
- Empty stoma losses according to individual neonate; this is done by removing the clip at the bottom of the bag, emptying and then re-placing clip tightly.
- Depending on the condition of the neonate and the stoma, the volume of output and other obstacles to bag adhesion, acceptable time intervals for stoma bag change may vary

(continued)

- After initial formation, the stoma will decrease in size, so it will be necessary to re-measure the stoma size as each new stoma bag is applied
- Angle the bag to encourage the contents to drain away from the stoma
- Consider oral sucrose for pain/discomfort management, pacifier for non-nutritive sucking and holding the neonate during stoma bag changing and care
- Refer/liaise and formulate stoma care plan with stoma nurse specialist for advice on bags, skin care and use of adjuncts such as any liquid barrier film and frequency of changing stoma bag

Documentation
- All stoma losses – colour, consistency and indication of amount ˙
- Complete stoma care plan and assessment
- If stoma losses are fluid, the volume in millilitres should be measured and recorded

Parental considerations
- Inform parents about and involve them in the care of their neonate's stoma. If discharged home, careful discharge planning will be required. This will include:
  - Parental teaching, assessment of parental competence to provide stoma care, supply of stoma appliances for discharge, arranging GP provision of stoma appliances in the community and support at home

 Remember standard precautions when performing stoma care including careful hand washing, use of gloves and aprons along with correct disposal of bags and stoma losses.

Check local guidance on stoma care

References: Patwardan et al. (2001); Waller (2008)

Fluid therapy and feeding the surgical neonate

Due to compromise to the bowel from surgery, surgical neonates have specific care needs with regard to fluid requirements and feeding regimes.

Figure 2.39 Fluid therapy and feeding the surgical neonate – DIAGRAM

Fluid requirements: Fluids (maintenance) are restricted in the immediate post-operative period for varying lengths of time due to the effects of anaesthesia and potential for overload. Increase as condition/recovery allows

Fluid replacement: Output lost from the bowel should be measured (from gastric or stoma losses that are discarded or insensible loss via an abdominal wall defect)

Replace losses with IV fluids (usually saline with potassium) as extra to maintenance either on a 'ml for ml' basis OR when losses reach a certain threshold agreed by the unit team

Feeding: Resume feeds when the bowel is able to tolerate and has recovered from surgery

Feeding readiness: Meconium or stool passing, bowel sounds, reduced/absent nasogastric losses that are clear

Milk: Feed preferably breast milk or, if required, special hydrolyzed formula that contains pre-digested protein for enhanced absorption and tolerance

Specific cases

In short gut when significant bowel has been resected, long-term absorption may be affected

Long-term/home TPN may be required with trophic 'priming' of the bowel via small amounts of milk (may be continuous)

Gastrostomy feeding may be required

Remember standard precautions when performing any practice relating to milk preparation and IV fluid therapy.

Check local guidance on feeding the surgical neonate

Compromise to the bowel may persist for a significant period depending on the quality of bowel resected or the post-operative response.

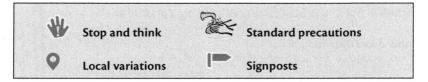

Stop and think   Standard precautions

Local variations   Signposts

Always ensure infection control and prevention is a central consideration in the pre-operative preparation of the surgical neonate as well as in the post-operative recovery stage.

The space below can be used to record any local variations and practice points specific to your own unit.

Surgical nursing practice: Glossary of surgical conditions

Abdominal distention: Air or fluid accumulates in the abdomen causing its outward expansion.

Cleft lip and/or palate: A type of clefting congenital deformity caused by abnormal facial development during the first trimester of fetal growth.

Congenital diaphragmatic hernia: Congenital defect involving an opening in the diaphragm, the large muscle that separates the chest and abdomen. Abdominal organs can move through the opening into the chest cavity.

Duodenal atresia: The congenital absence or complete closure of the lumen of the duodenum at some point along its length.

Exomphalos: A congenital anomaly where there is a herniation (protrusion) of the abdominal contents into the umbilical cord, which presents outside of the abdomen.

Gastric decompression: A procedure where a wide bore, short, nasogastric tube is used to remove the contents of the stomach including air (to decompress the stomach).

Gastro-oesophageal reflux: A condition where the stomach contents regurgitate back up into the lower oesophagus caused by a weak lower oesophageal sphincter (muscle).

Gastroschisis: Birth defect involving an opening in the abdominal wall, through which the abdominal organs bulge out without any sac or covering.

Hernia: Part of the body that is displaced and protrudes through the wall of the cavity containing it, for example, in the intestine.

Imperforate anus: A congenital defect of the anus where there is partial or complete obstruction of the anal opening.

Intestinal obstruction: Partial or complete blockage of the bowel that prevents the contents of the intestine from passing through.

Intussusception: Inversion of one portion of the intestine within another. Leads to acute intestinal obstruction.

Hirschprung's disease: Also known as *congenital aganglionic megacolon*, this is an abnormality in which certain nerve fibres are absent in segments of the bowel, resulting in intestinal obstruction.

Malrotation: A congenital anomaly of rotation of the mid-gut. As a result, the small bowel is found predominantly on the right side of the abdomen.

Meconium ileus: Congenital intestinal obstruction by thick meconium that fails to be passed.

Necrotizing enterocolitis (NEC): A disease process involving transmural necrosis and bacterial invasion of the bowel wall. The most commonly affected site is the terminal ileum, but any part of the bowel from stomach to rectum can be affected.

Oesophageal atresia (OA) with or without tracheoesophageal fistula (TOF): OA is where there is a blind end of the oesophagus and failure to join the stomach. TOF is a joining between the trachea and the oesophagus which can occur with OA.

Perforation: The penetration of a body part through accident or disease.

Pyloric stenosis: Narrowing of the pyloric sphincter (muscle) that blocks the passage of milk from the stomach into the duodenum.

Short gut: Otherwise known as short bowel syndrome. A malabsorption disorder caused by the surgical removal

of a large part of the small intestine, leaving a significantly small section.

Volvulus: An obstruction caused by twisting of the intestine leading to acute intestinal obstruction.

Surgical nursing practice: References

Brasher, C., Gafsous, B., Dugue, S., Thiollier, A., Kinderf, J., Nivoche, Y., and Dahmani, S. (2014). Postoperative pain management in children and infants: An update. *Pediatric Drugs.* 1–12.

de la Hunt, M.N. (2006). The acute abdomen in the newborn. *Seminars in Fetal and Neonatal Medicine.* 11 (3): 191–197.

Dickson, E. and Smith, C. (2006). Postoperative care of neonates. *Infant.* 2 (5): 178–182.

Harrell-Bean, H. and Klell, C. (2006). Neonatal ostomies. *JOGNN.* 12 (3): 69–73s.

Holland, A.J. and Fitzgerald, D.A. (2010). Oesophageal atresia and tracheo-oesophageal fistula: Current management strategies and complications. *Paediatric Respiratory Reviews.* 11 (2): 100–107.

Johnson, P.R.V. (2005). Oesophageal atresia. *Infant.* 1 (5): 163–167.

Kelly, A., Liddell, M., and Davis, C. (2008). The nursing care of the surgical neonate. *Seminars in Pediatric Surgery.* 17: 290–296.

Leeuwen, L. and Fitzgerald, D.A. (2014). Congenital diaphragmatic hernia. *Journal of Paediatrics and Child Health.* 50 (9): 667–793. DOI: 10.1111/jpc.12508.

Lund, C.H. and Berrios, M. (2007). Gastroschisis; incidence, complications and clinical management in the neonatal intensive care unit. *Journal of Perinatal and Neonatal Nursing.* 21 (1): 63–68.

Patwardhan, N., Kiely, E.M., Drake, D.P., Spitz, L., and Pierro, A. (2001). Colostomy for anorectal anomalies: High incidence of complications. *J Pediatr Surg.* 36 (5): 795–798.

Rogers, V. (2003). Managing preemie stomas: more than just the pouch. *Journal of Wound, Ostomy and Continence Nursing.* 30 (2): 100–110.

Royal College of Nursing (2011). *Transferring children to and from theatre.* London: RCN. http://www.rcn.org.uk/__data/assets/pdf_file/0003/395760/004127.pdf

Waller, M. (2008). Paediatric stoma care nursing in the UK and Ireland. *British Journal of Nursing.* 17 (17): S25.

Thermal care and transportation of the neonate

This chapter covers the following two topics under 'T'; Thermal care of the neonate and Transportation.

The thermal environment

As soon as a neonate is born, they are exposed to a significantly cooler extra-uterine environment and so thermal care is a vital consideration from the moment they are born. All neonates, due to their physiological immaturity, are predisposed to heat loss through various means and this vulnerability is even greater in the preterm neonate (Turnbull and Petty, 2013a, 2013b). Hypothermia can affect many other physiological systems and can be avoided by simple, fundamental measures that limit heat loss where possible (McCall et al., 2010, 2014) including incubator care (see Figure 2.40) and sound attention to the neutral thermal environment (NTE).

> Related topics. See also *Assessment* since temperature taking is an integral component of the overall assessment of the neonate. In addition, refer to *The three Hs* to see the significance of providing sound thermal care at birth for adaptation to extra-uterine life. Finally, *Kangaroo care* or skin-to-skin holding requires consideration in view of a strategy to prevent heat loss in the neonate.

Thermal care in the neonatal unit

Tables 2.35 and 2.36 and Figures 2.42 and 2.43 address various aspects of the thermal environment and related neonatal care.

Figure 2.40 Incubator

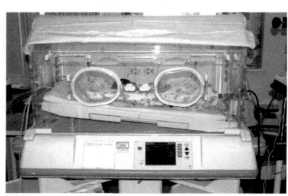

BAPM guidelines for the minimum central temperature of a neonate on admission to the neonatal unit from labour ward or other, is 36°C (BAPM, 2005). It is important to be mindful of admission temperatures to avoid adverse effects of hypothermia. See *The three Hs.*

Table 2.35   Heat loss methods and related thermal care – SUMMARY TABLE

Sources of heat loss	Preventive measures
Conduction **(Direct contact with cool surface)**	Warmed blankets or towels
	Hat
	Heated mattress
	Warmed IV solutions and gases
Convection **(Cool air currents)**	Room temperature for delivery should be 26°C (BAPM, 2005), neonatal unit 20–26°C and after discharge home, 18°C (Prevention of Cot Death Guidelines)
	Pre-warm Incubator – Figure 2.40
	Keep neonate covered
Radiation **(Heat radiating towards a cooler surface not in direct contact)**	Radiant warmer/Babytherm®
	Wrap neonate
	Warm room
Evaporation **(Heat loss through water vapour from wet skin)**	Heated, humidified inspired gases and body humidification (See Figure 2.43)
	Plastic bags/wrap (<28–30 weeks) – see Figure 2.41

 Standard precautions apply such as use of clean incubators, changing these according to local guidelines and hand washing before any thermal care.

 Observe local guidance for thermal care devices and their use.

References: Turnbull and Petty (2013a); McCall et al. (2014)

Figure 2.41 Preterm neonate in plastic bag

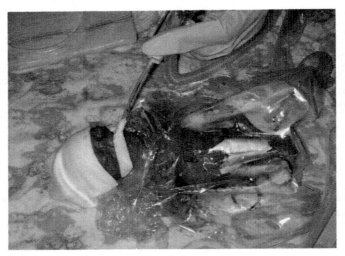

Figure 2.42 Methods of keeping neonates warm through dependency levels – DIAGRAM

Early care/birth

Term:/Well neonate: Dry, wrap and hat, skin to skin

Preterm: <28–30 weeks: Plastic bag and hat under radiant heater, transfer to humidified incubator as soon as possible

Admission to NNU 1

Closed, double-walled, pre-warmed incubator with humidity

Servo OR manual control*

Admission to NNU 2

Open overhead heater/'Babytherm' used for ease of access (e.g. surgical neonate or procedures)

Transition from incubator care 1: Heated mattress

Heat from a gel or water-filled, heated mattress

Transition from incubator care 2:

Bassinette (with or without heat shield)

Final transition to open cot: depends on unit guidelines and individual assessment of readiness (approx. 1.6 kg) (New et al., 2011)

 Observe local guidance

✋ *Servo is 'baby controlled' when a probe placed on the neonate's body (axilla or abdominal area) controls the temperature setting and heat delivered in order to maintain a desired temperature. Manual control is when the carer/user changes the delivered heat according to neonatal temperature readings at intervals (Allen, 2011).

The neutral thermal environment (NTE)

Wherever they are cared for, any newborn baby/neonate should be nursed in a neutral thermal environment (NTE). It is important therefore that the ambient environmental temperature is considered carefully, for example when preparing an incubator for a neonatal admission. Incubator care, providing both heat and humidity is the optimum method of providing a NTE in the first instance at a time when thermal control is limited. Age, gestation, weight and central body temperature must be considered in order to set the desired incubator temperature (Gardner et al, 2015).

Table 2.36   Guide to setting incubator temperatures – SUMMARY TABLE

Weight \ Age	Up to 24 hours	1-7 days	1-2 weeks	2-4 weeks	4-6 weeks	>6 weeks
Less than 1.5 kg	34–35	33–34	33.5–34	33–33.5	32.5–33	30–32
1.5 to 2.5 kg	33.5–34.5	32.5–33.5	32–32.5	31.5–32	30–31.5	n/a
Greater than 2.5 kg / term	32.5	32	31.5	30	n/a	n/a

N.B: Temperatures are in degrees Celsius and are *suggested* averages. A range (plus or minus 0.5 -1 degree above or below) should be considered. Incubator temperatures should be adjusted according to the neonate's recorded central temperature.

✋ After a neonate is transferred from an incubator to an open cot, one should be mindful of the ambient room temperatures. Table 2.35 outlines the recommendations for these within both hospital and the home environment.

Humidification

Generally, a neonate <28–30 weeks, <1 kg in weight and in the first 7–10 days should be nursed in 50–90% relative humidity via a closed incubator such as the Ohmeda 'Giraffe'® or similar to provide their optimum NTE.

Figure 2.43 Humidification in thermal care – FLOW CHART

Place neonate into a plastic bag at birth under radiant heater until transferred to a warmed humidified incubator (Kent and Williams 2008; Rohana et al., 2011). Minimize the length of time spent under a radiant heater and move the neonate into a closed incubator as soon as possible

Humidify the incubator
Up to 85–90% humidity may be required but the range is 50–90% depending on neonate's temperature as well as *sodium/fluid balance

After 14–21 days, assess temperature, *fluid and sodium balance and discontinue humidification following agreement with the neonatal team. *Remember that humidification not only helps prevent transepidermal heat loss but also that of water through the skin. Sodium imbalance can arise (high sodium) if water losses are significant. (Sinclair et al., 2009).

Due to the moist environment as a consequence of humidity, be mindful of this when changing incubators. Use sterile water to refill humidity chamber in the incubator.

Observe local guidance for humidification procedure

A neonate's temperature, along with fluid and electrolyte status, should be monitored when administering humidity and considering when to stop, until skin has keratinized (Turnbull and Petty, 2012).

Stop and think   Standard precautions

 Local variations   Signposts

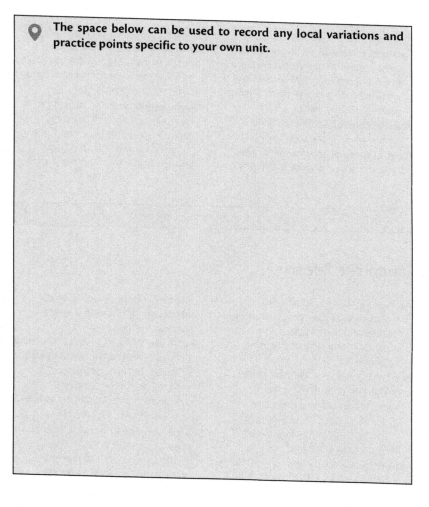 Always apply principles of good hand washing when handling a neonate to take their temperature.

The space below can be used to record any local variations and practice points specific to your own unit.

Thermal care: Glossary

Bassinette: A small cradle type cot for newborns prior to being nursed in a cot.

Conduction: Heat is transmitted or lost through direct contact.

Convection: Heat is transmitted or lost through circulating air currents.

Evaporation: Heat is transmitted and lost as water becomes a vapour.

Hyperthermia: Body temperature above the normal range.

Hypothermia: Body temperature below 35°C.

Incubator: Neonates who are low birth weight, preterm or are cold are placed in a pre-warmed, double-walled and enclosed crib to enable them to keep warm or to gain heat.

Manual control: Setting ambient temperature by the user/nurse/carer.

Neutral thermal environment: The environmental temperature at which a neonate uses minimal rates of oxygen consumption and expends the least energy.

Radiation: The transfer of heat energy through space.

Relative humidity: A measure of how much water vapour is in a gas or in the atmosphere compared to its capacity to hold water vapour. It is measured as a percentage.

Radiant warmer: Open bed with an overhead radiant heat source to warm the neonate.

Servo control: Setting the ambient temperature using a probe on the neonate's skin, which regulates the air temperature accordingly.

Thermoregulation: The capacity to maintain homeostasis (balance) between heat production and heat loss in order to sustain the body temperature within a normal range.

 The Glossary for *The three Hs* is also relevant for this topic

Thermal care: References

Allen, K. (2011). Neonatal thermal care: A discussion of two incubator modes for neonatal thermoregulation. A care study. *Journal of Neonatal Nursing.* 17 (2): 43–48.

British Association of Perinatal Medicine (2005). *Early care of the newborn infant. Statement on current level of evidence.* http://www.bapm.org/publications/documents/guidelines/RDS_position-statement.pdf

Gardner, SL, Carter, BS, Enzman-Hines, MI & Hernandez, JA. (2015). Merenstein &

Gardner's Handbook of Neonatal Intensive Care (8th ed). St Louis/London; Mosby.

Kent, A. and Williams, J. (2008). Increasing ambient operating theatre temperature and wrapping in polyethylene improves admission temperature in premature infants. *Journal of Paediatrics and Child Health.* 44: 325–331.

McCall, E.M., Alderdice, F., Halliday, H.L., Jenkins, J.G., and Vohra, S. (2010). Interventions to prevent hypothermia at birth in preterm and/or low birthweight infants. *Cochrane Database of Systematic Reviews.* Issue 3. Art. No.: CD004210.

McCall, E., Alderdice, F., Halliday, H., Johnston, L., and Vohra, S. (2014). Challenges of minimising heat loss at birth: A narrative overview of evidence-based thermal care interventions. *Newborn and Infant Nursing Reviews.* 14 (2): 56–63.

New, K., Flenady, V., and Davies, M.W. (2011). Transfer of preterm infants from incubator to open cot at lower versus higher body weight. *Cochrane Database of Systematic Reviews.* Issue 9. Art. No.: CD004214.

Rohana, J., Khairina, W., Boo, N.Y., and Shareena, I. (2011). Reducing hypothermia in preterm infants with polyethylene wrap. *Pediatr Int.* 53 (4): 468–474.

Sinclair, L., Crisp, J., and Sinn, J. (2009). Variability in incubator humidity practices in the management of preterm infants. *Journal of Paediatrics and Child Health.* 45: 535–540.

Turnbull, V. and Petty, J. (2013a). Understanding evidence-based thermal care in the low birth weight neonate: Part 1: An overview of principles and current practice. *Nursing Children and Young People.* 25 (2): 18–22.

Turnbull, V and Petty, J. (2013b) Evidence-based thermal care of low birth weight neonates. Part 2: family-centred care principles. *Nursing Children and Young People.* 25 (3): 26–29.

Transportation of the neonate

This section focuses on neonatal transportation. It is vital that access to a tertiary neonatal intensive care unit (NICU) is available for all unstable newborn infants. Maternal antenatal transfer provides more favourable outcomes for ill newborns and adverse events have been associated with *ex utero* (Towers et al., 2000; Ratnavel, 2013). However, some neonates will inevitably need to be transported acutely to NICUs (Chang et al., 2008). In reverse, it is equally important to have a good system in place to facilitate their transfer back to the hospital of booking. Boxes 2.54 and 2.55 deal with stabilization and transfer preparation.

> ▌➡
> Related topics. *See Assessment* for the principles of stabilization following birth and thereafter in the neonatal unit.

Stabilizing for transfer

Stabilization of the sick neonate prior to transporting them is essential to ensure best outcomes. While waiting for the retrieval team, to prepare for transfer, a checklist for stabilization is useful. Box 2.54 below contains some of the main points to consider.

> ✋
> **Time taken to stabilize a neonate and optimize their condition is time well spent prior to transporting them to another centre.**

Box 2.54   Stabilization prior to transfer – CHECKLIST

Airway management • establish a patent airway • evaluate the need for oxygen, or an artificial airway • security of the airway – (ETT) must be secure to prevent intra-transport dislodgement • chest X-ray – to check position of the ETT

Breathing • the need for intra-transport ventilation has to be assessed • oxygenation • blood gases • tachypnoea and expected respiratory fatigue • recurrent apnoea episodes • consider if it is safer to intubate for transfer

Circulation • heart rate and perfusion (capillary refill) are good indicators of CVS status • blood pressure • intravenous access (at least 2 cannulae) • if dehydrated, the neonate must be rehydrated before leaving

(continued)

Communication · good communication between the different teams will help better coordination of the transfer · inform the receiving specialist unit · patient details · history/physical findings/provisional diagnosis/investigations · current management and status of the baby · mode of transport · use of SBAR – ▐➤ See *Communication*

Drugs as required · antibiotics · analgesia/sedation, especially if neonate is intubated · inotropes · vitamin K

Documentation · history including antenatal and birth history/physical findings/diagnosis · input/output charts · investigation results/X-rays · parents' contact telephone numbers

Environment · neutral thermal environment · optimal temperature for the neonate (axilla) · prevention of heat loss · incubator heated and transwarmer ready unless passive cooling is required. ▐➤ See *Neurological care*

Equipment · ▐➤ See Box 2.55. Check all equipment

Fluid therapy · resuscitation fluid, maintenance fluid, other ongoing or anticipated losses in the surgical neonate, e.g. intestinal obstruction, gastroschisis

Gastric decompression · an orogastric tube will be required in surgical neonates with hourly aspiration and free flow of the gastric contents

Immediately before departure

CHECK clinical condition and vital signs, positioning, pain and stress levels, secure the neonate and all tubes, function of equipment

Re-communicate with receiving unit about current status and expected time of arrival

PARENTS – include as part of stabilization process and consider their needs ▐➤ See *Psychosocial care of the family*

⬤ Check local guidance on referral processes for transfer and stabilization procedures

References: Kendall et al (2010); Singh et al (2010); Chawla et al (2011); van den Berg and Lindh (2011); Harrison and McKechnie (2012); Helder et al., (2012).

Preparing for transportation

Even for staff who are not part of a dedicated team, transfers may still occur within the hospital to and from the delivery suite, X-ray dept. and other locations. In addition, non-urgent back transfers may also be carried out by neonatal staff. A transport incubator checklist can therefore be useful to promote safety and preparation for this care.

Box 2.55   Checking the transport incubator – CHECKLIST

Transport incubator
- Check function before leaving the hospital
- Ventilator working without any leaks, gives pressure
- Monitors: cardiorespiratory and pulse oximeter
- Infusion pumps with adequately charged batteries
- Suction device functions properly
- Oxygen cylinders – ensure adequacy for the whole journey

Equipment
- Intubation and ventilation equipment and ETTs of varying sizes (laryngoscope, Magill forceps, batteries with spares)
- Manual resuscitation (BVM) bags and masks of appropriate sizes are available and in working order
- Suction apparatus and catheters/tubing
- Oxygen tubing
- Anticipated medication and water for dilution and injection
- IV fluids, giving sets. Pre-draw fluids or medication into syringes if required
- Intravenous cannulae of various sizes
- Needles of different sizes
- Syringes and tubing
- Suture material
- Adhesive tape, scissors
- Gloves, gauze, swabs
- Stethoscope
- Thermometer
- Nasogastric tube
- Transwarmer mattress
- Chest clamps (if water seal chest drain is present)

Ensure the transport incubator and all equipment is cleaned according to local policy

Check local guidance on checking procedures

As for any essential equipment, being familiar with the presence and working of the transport incubator maximizes safety.

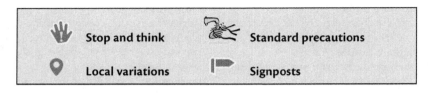

Stop and think   Standard precautions

Local variations   Signposts

Always apply principles of infection control even when a neonate is being stabilized for transfer out and during any transportation.

The space below can be used to record any local variations and practice points specific to your own unit.

Transportation: Glossary

Back transfer: Transfer back to the original 'home' unit.

Ex-utero transfer: The transportation of a neonate following delivery from a referral unit to a receiving unit.

In utero transfer: The transportation of a high-risk pregnant mother following referral to a centre where she will give birth. Primary emphasis should always remain on prenatal diagnosis and subsequent *in utero* (i.e. maternal) transfer whenever possible.

Tertiary centre: Referral centre for further management.

Transport incubator: A portable version of an incubator combined with full ventilation and monitoring capability to transfer sick and/or small neonates between units.

Transwarmer: A gel-filled, thermostable disposable mattress that provides up to two hours of warming when cold stress is a concern.

Transportation: References

Chang, A.S.M., Berry, A., and Sivasangari S. (2008). Specialty teams for neonatal transport to neonatal intensive care units for prevention of morbidity and mortality (Protocol). *Cochrane Database of Systematic Reviews.* Issue 4. Art. No.: CD007485.

Chawla, S., Amaram, A., Gopal, S.P., and Natarajan, G. (2011). Safety and efficacy of Trans-warmer mattress for preterm neonates: Results of a randomized controlled trial. *Journal of Perinatology.* 31 (12): 780–784.

Harrison, C. and McKechnie, L. (2012). How comfortable is neonatal transport? *Acta Paediatrica.* 101 (2): 143–147.

Helder, O.K., Verweij, J.C., and van Staa, A. (2012). Transition from neonatal intensive care unit to special care nurseries: Experiences of parents and nurses. *Pediatric Critical Care Medicine.* 13 (3): 305–311.

Kendall, G.S., Kapetanakis, A., Ratnavel, N., Azzopardi, D., and Robertson, N.J. (2010). Passive cooling for initiation of therapeutic hypothermia in neonatal encephalopathy. *Arch Dis Child Fetal Neonatal Ed.* 95: F408–F412.

Ratnavel, N. (2013). Evaluating and Improving neonatal transfer services. *Early Human Development.* 89 (11): 851–853.

Singh, A., Duckett, J., Newton, T., and Watkinson, M. (2010) Improving neonatal unit admission temperatures in preterm babies: Exothermic mattresses, polythene bags or a traditional approach? *Journal of Perinatology.* 30: 45–49.

Towers, C.V., Bonebrake, R., Padilla, G., and Rumney, P. (2000). The effect of transport on the rate of severe intraventricular haemorrhage in very low birth weight infants. *Obstet Gynecol.* 95 (2): 291–295.

van den Berg, J. and Lindh, V. (2011). Back transport of infants to community hospitals: 12 years' experience of an intervention to prepare parents for their infants' transfer from neonatal intensive care to community hospital. *Journal of Neonatal Nursing.* 17 (3): 116–125.

Umbilical care and catheters

This chapter addresses the care issues around use and care of the umbilical cord.

In the healthy term or preterm neonate at birth, evidence supports the recommendation to leave the cord for at least one minute prior to clamping and cutting (Rabe et al., 2012; Duley and Batey, 2013; McDonald et al., 2013). Once clamped and cut, the cord is then kept clean and is observed until the stump separates. In the sick or high-risk neonate who requires admission after birth to neonatal care, the cord is clamped and cut immediately leaving a long stump, which is then catheterized. Box 2.56 deals specifically with the care issues around umbilical vessel catheterization.

> Related topics. See also *Blood and blood taking* for information relevant to arterial line sampling, *Cardiovascular care*, for information on monitoring blood pressure and calibration of an arterial line and *Hygiene needs* which covers cleaning of the umbilicus.

> **The timing of cord clamping is open to debate and differing opinions. This is an area of practice with ever-emerging evidence in relation to optimum timing for well and at-risk/sick neonates.**
>
> **Any umbilical catheter has associated risks which should be observed on at least an hourly basis and documented. Catheters should be removed if any concern arises (Furdon et al., 2006).**

Box 2.56   Umbilical catheter care overview – CHECKLIST

Use of umbilical cord at birth

- At birth, the cord can be used for blood sampling and once cut, the umbilical vein can be used for catheterization when emergency resuscitation drugs are required
- In an unstable, sick neonate who requires admission to intensive care, both an umbilical venous catheter and an arterial catheter can be inserted (UVC/UAC)

UVC: For fluid and drug administration.
UAC: For arterial monitoring and blood sampling.

(continued)

Positions for umbilical catheters

- There are two potential positions for the UAC. These are described as 'high' or 'low' and confirmed on chest X-ray (MacDonald and Ramasethu, 2002)
- The high position is at the level of thoracic vertebral bodies T6–T9 above the diaphragm. The low position is at the level of lumbar vertebral bodies L3–L4. Both avoid points that may interfere with perfusion to vital organs

References: Barrington (1999); Sritipsukho and Sritipsukho (2007); van Schuppen et al. (2013)

Care of UAC/UVCs

- UACs: The same principles apply as for care of arterial lines in general (see *Cardiovascular system care* Boxes 2.19a and 2.19b) and blood sampling from arterial lines (see *Blood and blood taking* Box 2.15)
- The umbilical vein and artery are central vessels and so care must be taken to avoid potential complications such as bleeding, reduced blood flow to the limbs and blockage.
- Neonates with UACs/UVCs are not placed prone
- Lower limbs need to be closely observed for adequate perfusion and signs of compromise to blood flow
- The stump should be well secured and observed for bleeding and redness/infection
- Ensure UAC has heparinised saline running through at all times according to local policy. UVCs will be kept open by maintenence fluids infusing.
- Remove the catheters when vessels are no longer patent or complications/concerns arise

 Ensure thorough hand washing and wear gloves when handling umbilical catheters for any purpose.

 Observe local guidance on the timing of cord clamping, catheterization of the umbilical vessels and the subsequent care thereafter

Stop and think		**Standard precautions**	
Local variations		**Signposts**	

 Strict adherence to standard precautions is essential during any umbilical access to prevent the introduction of infection via this route which gives central access to the cardiovascular system.

The space below can be used to record any local variations and practice points specific to your own unit.

Umbilical catheters: Glossary

Umbilical catheter: Thin tube inserted into an umbilical artery or vein that can be used to sample blood (umbilical arterial catheter) or give fluids, drugs, nutrients or blood (umbilical venous catheter).

Umbilical cord: The connection between the placenta and the fetus in pregnancy, which is clamped and cut at birth. The umbilical cord has two arteries and one vein.

Umbilical catheters: References

Barrington, K.J. (1999). Umbilical artery catheters in the newborn: Effects of heparin. *Cochrane Database of Systematic Reviews.* Issue 1. Art. No.: CD000507. DOI: 10.1002/14651858. CD000507. Updated 2009.

Duley, L. and Batey, N. (2013). Optimal timing of umbilical cord clamping for term and preterm babies. *Early Human development.* 89 (11): 905–908.

Furdon, S.A., Horgan, M.J., Bradshaw, W.T., and Clark, D.A. (2006). Nurses' guide to early detection of umbilical arterial catheter complications in infants. *Advances in Neonatal Care.* 6 (5): 257–260.

MacDonald, M.G. and Ramasethu, J. (2002). Umbilical artery catheterization. In: *Atlas of Procedures in Neonatology.* 3rd ed. Philadelphia: Lippincott Williams and Wilkins.

McDonald, S.J., Middleton, P., Dowswell, T., and Morris, P.S. (2013). Effect of timing of umbilical cord clamping of term infants on maternal and neonatal outcomes. *Cochrane Database of Systematic Reviews.* Issue 7. Art. No.: CD004074.

Rabe, H., Diaz-Rossello, J.L., Duley, L. and Dowswell, T. (2012). Effect of timing of umbilical cord clamping and other strategies to influence placental transfusion at preterm birth on maternal and infant outcomes. *Cochrane Database of Systematic Reviews.* Issue 8. Art. No.: CD003248.

Sritipsukho, S. and Sritipsukho, P. (2007). Simple and accurate formula to estimate umbilical arterial catheter length of high placement. *J Med Assoc Thai.* 90 (9): 1793–1797.

van Schuppen, J., Onland, W., and van Rijn, R. (2013). *Neonatal Chest X-Ray; Lines and tubes.* http://www.radiologyassistant.nl/en/p526bd2e468b8c/neonatal-chest-x-ray.html

Vomiting and reflux

This chapter focuses on the subject of vomiting and reflux in the neonate.

Many neonates vomit at some time. In most cases this is unimportant. However, there are circumstances when the type of vomiting *is* important and therefore having a guide to this may be useful to inform practice. Table 2.37 covers an overview of the types of vomiting and implications for practice.

> Related topics. See also *Gastrointestinal care and feeding* and *Surgical care practices.*

Table 2.37	A guide to the neonate who is vomiting – SUMMARY TABLE
Key messages	

- Most neonates vomit; in most cases this is insignificant, for example, 'posits' that are small but frequent
- Most worrying is the presence of blood or bile
- Any neonate who is sick, has deteriorated, who fails to thrive, has reflux, bilious or projectile vomiting is a cause for concern

Type of vomit	Practice points
With blood	May have swallowed maternal blood during labour or the neonate may be bleeding: e.g. clotting deficiency, stress ulceration caused by steroids or indomethacin. Observe closely, document and ascertain cause
Bilious vomiting	Green vomit. Obstruction always presumed until otherwise confirmed. Pass wide bore nasogastric tube and aspirate. May need a surgical referral (Godbole and Stringer, 2002)
Projectile	May be a sign of duodenal obstruction or pyloric stenosis if after 2–3 weeks of life. As above, treat as for surgical emergency if these conditions are suspected
The neonate who is unwell	A sign of infection or metabolic disorder. Observe closely, document and ascertain cause

(continued)

Table 2.37   Continued

Type of vomit	Practice points
Significant gastro-oesophageal reflux with or without failure to thrive	Effortless vomiting especially when lying flat. Elevate head of bed, position neonate in prone or left lateral position*, thicken feeds and feed more frequently with smaller volumes. Antacid and/or anticholinergic drugs. Minimal handling after feeding. Observe for potential aspiration
	*The prone or left lateral position reduces acid reflux. As these positions increase the risk of cot death, they should only be utilized on the neonatal unit where cardio-respiratory monitoring is in place. Parents should be advised to place infants in the supine position when discharged home *References*: Valappil and Ramesh (2011); Chen et al. (2013); Corvaglia et al. (2013)
With concurrent diarrhoea	Possible gastroenteritis. Requires investigation into cause of infection, stool specimens, rehydration, intravenous *if necessary*

Any bilious vomiting should be treated as an emergency and referral is time critical for immediate surgical review (Mohinuddin et al., 2012; Radwan et al., 2012).

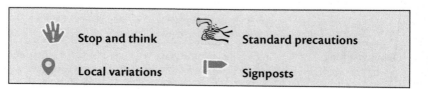

	Stop and think		Standard precautions
	Local variations		Signposts

Always wear gloves when handling any bodily fluid such as vomit or gastric aspirates.

The space below can be used to record any local variations and practice points specific to your own unit.

Vomiting and reflux: Glossary

Posit: Small quantity of regurgitated curdled milk.

Reflux: The movement of the stomach contents back up into the oesophagus.

Vomit: The ejection of matter from the stomach through the mouth.

Vomiting and reflux: References

Chen, S.S., Tzeng, Y.L., Gau, B.S., Kuo, P.C., and Chen, J.Y. (2013). Effects of prone and supine positioning on gastric residuals in preterm infants: A time series with cross-over study. *International Journal of Nursing Studies.* 50 (11): 1459–1467.

Corvaglia, L., Martini, S., and Faldella, G. (2013). Gastro-oesophageal reflux: Pathogenesis, symptoms, diagnostic and therapeutic management. *Early Human Development.* 89: S18–S19.

Godbole, P. and Stringer, M.D. (2002). Bilious vomiting in the newborn: How often is it pathological? *Journal of Pediatric Surgery.* 37 (6): 909–911.

Mohinuddin, S.M., Sakhuja, P., Flemming, P., Bermundo, B., Mohidin, R., Ratnavel, N., and Kempley, S. (2012). Term neonates with bilious vomiting – Should they be considered as time critical transfers to the surgical centre? *Arch Dis Child.* 97: A106.

Radwan, R., Ram, A.D., and Huddart, S.N. (2012). A few hours from disaster. *BMJ: British Medical Journal.* 345: e4441 doi: http://dx.doi.org/10.1136/bmj.e4441

Valappil, S., and Ramesh, C. (2011). A survey on management of gastro oesophageal reflux in infants, across the United Kingdom. *Pediatric Research.* 70: 840.

Weight

This penultimate chapter in Part 2 addresses the subject of weight as a valuable and commonplace parameter for growth in neonatal care.

Weights are measured and plotted for all neonates whether they are healthy or sick at varying intervals depending on need and the individual situation. Box 2.57, Figure 2.44 and Table 2.38 cover three areas: a guide to weight patterns, an overview of the terminology used to describe weight and how to distinguish between low birth weight and preterm neonates.

> Related topics. See also *Assessment* for consideration of weight as an important parameter within a holistic perspective. In addition, see *Gastrointestinal care and feeding* in relation to calculating feed volumes using weight along with importance of good nutrition for adequate weight gain.

> **Weight is an important and essential guide for fluid management on a daily basis in a sick neonate.**

Box 2.57   Guide to weight patterns and plotting – CHECKLIST

Understanding weight

- All newborns lose up to 10% of their birth weight within the first few days of life with weight gain commencing at 3–5 days (Wright and Parkinson, 2004; RCPCH, 2013)
- Weight is usually regained by 2 weeks (80% of all well newborns; RCPCH, 2013)
- Feeds, fluids and drugs are calculated on birth weight until this has been regained – after then, generally, calculations are on *current* weight
- Normal intrauterine growth is 10–15 g/kg/day although preterm neonates rarely achieve this (Tsang et al., 2006)
- Well term neonates should be weighed at 5 and 10 days. In the neonatal unit, however, neonates should be weighed every 24 hours if possible

(continued)

- Length and head circumference are also important growth parameters to measure once weekly in conjunction with weight, as these are indices of skeletal and organ growth, whereas weight can be influenced by fluid changes and fat deposition

Understanding plotting

- Plot neonatal weight/height/head circumference on recommended growth/centile chart according to their gestation born (RCPCH, 2009a, 2009b, 2013). There are three possible charts: an infancy chart for those born 37–42 weeks gestation, a preterm neonate chart for between 32 and 37 weeks gestation and a low birth weight chart for those born less than 32 weeks
- Follow the guidelines produced by RCPCH (2009a, 2009b)
- Birth is day 0
- No line exists for the 1st 2 weeks to allow for the normal weight loss
- If there is significant weight loss, or the neonate is still below birth weight at 2 weeks, calculate % weight loss:

$$\frac{\text{Weight loss (g)} \times 100}{\text{Birth Weight (g)}} = \% \text{ Weight lost}$$

- Weight loss of 10% or more needs careful assessment: this can indicate dehydration. No weight loss or gain in the early days indicates fluid overload.
- Monitoring of weight over time is important (McKie et al., 2006) – observe the centile corresponding with the measured weight and the progression thereafter
- Neonates commonly lose weight and change/drop centiles if they are sick and spend significant time in hospital. Similarly, centiles may increase. Nutritional management must consider these situations and be optimized appropriately. Accelerated growth should be avoided

  ⦿ Observe local guidance on agreed procedures for monitoring weight

---

Weight in line with gestation can be monitored during pregnancy by scanning in the second and third trimester. This may identify at-risk neonates prior to delivery.

Figure 2.44 Terminology used to understand birth weight – DIAGRAM

| Low birth weight (LBW) | • **LBW;** Low birth weight. <2.5 kg
• **VLBW;** Very low birth weight <1.5 kg
• **ELBW;** Extremely low birth weight <1 kg |

| Weight and gestational age | • **AGA;** Appropriate for gestational age – growth is as expected for gestation
• **SGA;** Small for gestational age; also called 'small for dates' – growth is less than expected for gestation (<10th centile)
• **LGA;** Large for gestational age – growth is more than expected for gestation, > 90th centile (e.g. macrosomia) |

| Intrauterine growth restriction (IUGR) | • **IUGR;** Intra uterine growth restriction. Growth that is not permitted to reach the maximum growth potential due to problems during pregnancy
• **Symmetrical IUGR;** Growth restriction that is proportional for both head and body: i.e. both are small and have remained so throughout pregnancy. Causes: genetic, chromosomal or congenital infection
• **Asymmetrical IUGR;** Growth restriction whereby head/brain growth is within expected norms but the body growth is reduced: i.e. head and body are disproportionate. Causes: poor placental function hindering transfer of nutrients and oxygen to the fetus |

References: WHO (2011); Smith et al. (2013); Ross (2013); Subramanian et al. (2014)

Table 2.38 Guide to distinguishing growth restricted and preterm neonates (<34 weeks) – SUMMARY TABLE

Differences		
Assessment feature	Preterm	IUGR
Physiological systems	Immature	Mature (as for term)
Airway and breathing	Surfactant deficiency and pulmonary immaturity/insufficiency	Lungs in alveolar stage of development and producing surfactant

(continued)

Table 2.38   Continued

	Differences	
Assessment feature	Preterm	IUGR
Gastrointestinal tract	Poor suck/swallow reflex. Unable to feed orally	Able to suck and swallow and feed normally. Often very hungry with lusty cry
Musculoskeletal system	Poor tone and flat, extended posture	Physiological flexion formed, good muscle tone, flexed limbs
Pinna of ear	No cartilage and floppy	Cartilage and formed
Nipple	Not raised	Raised
Sole of foot	Smooth	Creases evident
Skin	Red and shiny (very preterm) Fragile. Lacks keratin	Formed skin with keratin formed May be baggy due to reduced subcutaneous fat
	Similarities	
Weight	<2.5 kg	<2.5 kg
Thermoregulation	Poor thermal control	Poor thermal control
Blood glucose	Lack of glycogen reserves and at risk of hypoglycaemia	Lack of glycogen reserves and at risk of hypoglycaemia
Nutrition	Lack of nutritional reserves from pregnancy	Lack of nutritional reserves from pregnancy

> The neonate who is growth restricted has similar potential problems to the one born preterm but there are also some differences – it is important to understand the latter in order to guide management appropriately.

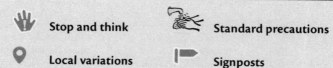

Stop and think   Standard precautions

Local variations   Signposts

The space below can be used to record any local variations and practice points specific to your own unit.

Weight: Glossary

Catch up: The weight of a neonate that was below expected norms, that subsequently increases or accelerates.

Centile or percentile: A value on a scale of one hundred that indicates the percent of a distribution that is equal to or below it (<a percentile score of 95 is a score equal to or better than 95 percent of the scores.)

Gestational age: Gestation at which a neonate is born between 23/24 weeks up to 40 weeks full term.

Growth chart: The chart used to plot a neonate's weight according to their age giving information on trends in weight over time and the relevant percentile.

Growth parameters: Measures used to assess growth; include weight, length and head circumference in the neonate.

Macrosomia: A condition in which a neonate is born with excessive birth weight, commonly due to maternal diabetes and may require delivery through caesarean section.

This glossary should be used in conjunction with Figure 2.44: terminology used to understand birth weight.

Weight: References

McKie, A., Young, D., MacDonald, P.D. (2006). Does monitoring newborn weight discourage breast feeding? *Arch Dis Child.* 91 (1): 44–46.

Ross, M.G. (2013) Fetal growth restriction. http://emedicine.medscape.com/article/261226-overview

Royal College of Paediatrics and Child Health (RCPCH) (2009a). *UK-WHO growth charts – Fact sheet 4 – Plotting and assessing newborn infants.*

Royal College of Paediatrics and Child Health (RCPCH) (2009b). *UK-WHO growth charts – Fact sheet 5 – Plotting preterm infants.*

Royal College of Paediatrics and Child Health (RCPCH). (2013). *UK-WHO 0–4 years growth chart resources.* http://www.rcpch.ac.uk/child-health/research-projects/uk-who-growth-charts/uk-who-growth-chart-resources-0-4-years/uk-who-0

Smith, J., Murphy, M., and Kandasamy, Y. (2013). The IUGR infant: A case study and associated problems with IUGR infants. *Journal of Neonatal Nursing.* 19 (2): 46–53.

Subramanian, S, Barton, A.M, and Montazami, S. (2014). Extremely Low Birthweight Infant. http://emedicine.medscape.com/article/979717-overview

Tsang, R.C., Lucas, A., Uauy, R., and Zlotkin, S. (2006). *Nutritional needs of the preterm infant: scientific basis and practical guidelines.* Baltimore: Williams & Wilkins.

World Health Organization (WHO) (2011). *Guidelines on optimal feeding of low birthweight infants in low- and middle-income countries.* Geneva: WHO.

Wright, C.M. and Parkinson, K.N. (2004). Postnatal weight loss in term infants: What is normal and do growth charts allow for it? *Arch Dis Child Fetal Neonatal Ed.* 89 (3):F254–F257.

X-rays and imaging

This final chapter in Part 2 outlines the different modes of imaging used in neonatal care for assessment and/or diagnosis.

X-rays and ultrasonography, for example, are frequently carried out in the neonatal unit, particularly in acute, intensive care and provide valuable information to add to our clinical assessment of respiratory and neurological status respectively. Table 2.39 offers a guide to imaging modes summarizing their use and nursing practice points.

> Related topics. See also *Assessment* since X-ray interpretation is a common and important part of a holistic approach. X-ray analysis is also used commonly to assess the effect of respiratory management (*Breathing*), surfactant administration (*Respiratory distress*) and to assist in the diagnosis of surgical conditions (*Surgical section*). Finally, ultrasound is commonplace to assess for and monitor IVH in the preterm neonate (*Neurological care*).

> Observation is important during any imaging, not only to ensure the neonate remains safe but also to ensure the optimum image is taken without artefact.

Table 2.39 Overview of X-rays and scanning in the neonatal unit –
SUMMARY TABLE

Procedure	Use	Practice points
X-ray	Chest: diagnosis of respiratory conditions, confirms lung collapse, consolidation or air leaks Determines line positions, e.g. peripherally inserted central catheters, umbilical catheters, nasogastric tubes, endotracheal tubes	During X-rays, the neonate needs to be aligned correctly, lie still and should be free of any factor that may cause artefact and inhibit proper interpretation

(continued)

Table 2.39   Continued

Procedure	Use	Practice points
	Abdomen: diagnosis of intestinal obstruction/ conditions and presence/ position of gas within the bowel	
Ultrasound	Head ultrasound: assessment of the neurological status of the neonate as well as diagnosis/grading of intraventricular haemorrhage (IVH) and periventricular leucomalacia (PVL)	Observe and assist with neonate's stress levels and exposure
	Information about immediate and long-term prognosis. A fast bedside examination	
	Echocardiogram: a heart ultrasound to visualize blood flow, direction and to diagnose cardiac compromise/PPHN	
	Hips: can diagnose congenital dysplasia of the hips	
CT scan (computer tomography) and MRI (magnetic resonance imaging)	Less common scans but are done for more detail when images of structure are necessary (e.g. long-term brain damage, following therapeutic cooling (MRI))	These require careful planning and transfer to X-ray department when clinically stable
Fluoroscopy	Barium studies	As above. Close assessment is necessary during the procedure
	Barium enema for investigation into lower intestinal obstruction	
	Barium swallow for investigation into upper intestine, i.e. for gastro-oesophageal reflux	
	Less common procedures may also be undertaken for cardiac investigations	

References: Arthur (2001); Beek and Groenendaal (2006); NHS NIPEP (2010); Mooneyham (2012)

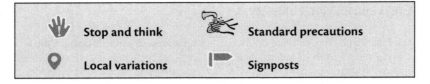

Stop and think

Standard precautions

Local variations

Signposts

The space below can be used to record any local variations and practice points specific to your own unit.

X-rays and imaging: Glossary

Artefact: Something observed on X-ray that is not naturally present or in the case of monitoring, may be caused by interference.

Computed tomography (CT or CAT scan): Computer-processed X-rays to produce tomographic images (virtual 'slices') of specific areas of the scanned object, allowing the user to see what is inside it.

Echocardiogram: A specialized form of ultrasound examination that is used to visualize the heart.

Fluoroscopy: Using a contrast medium to visualize moving images within the body.

Magnetic resonance imaging (MRI): Imaging technique that uses powerful magnets and computers to produce a detailed picture of tissue.

Ultrasonography (ultrasound scanning): Imaging technique that uses sound waves to make a picture of tissue, for example, the brain.

X-ray: Or radiograph. An image produced on a sensitive plate or film by radiation (energy that comes from a source and travels through some material).

X-rays and Imaging: References

Arthur, R. (2001). The neonatal chest X-ray. *Pediatric Respiratory Reviews*. 2: 311–323.

Beek, E. and Groenendaal, F. (2006). Neonatal brain US. Radiology assistant. Retrieved at http://www.radiologyassistant.nl/en/p440c93be7456f/neonatal-brain-us.html

Mooneyham, S. (2012). Diagnostic processes. In: C. Kenner and J. Lott (eds), *Comprehensive Neonatal Nursing Care (5th edition)*. New York: Springer.

NHS Newborn and Infant Physical Examination Programme. (2010). Ultrasound examination of the hips in screening for developmental dysplasia of the hips (DDH). http://newbornphysical.screening.nhs.uk/standards

Author's concluding comments

This book is intended to support bedside care of the neonate in the clinical setting. Clinical care is constantly evolving and we should be mindful of this as we care for our vulnerable neonatal population and their families. It is imperative that we keep up to date with changes and developments in clinical practice. Moreover, as stated in the introduction, certain areas of practice are particularly subject to regular change and debates will always exist in relation to best practice, for example; the timing of cord clamping at birth, operational thresholds to give blood transfusions and advances in ventilation support, to name but a few. The aim is that this book will also evolve as practices change in the future.

We must also be aware that the areas covered in this book have a theoretical background in which to delve further to enquire and learn more about the rationale for practice. The reader can undertake further reading through the references provided for each section and the recommended links for learning further about the underpinning theory. Further enquiry is important due to the nature of current and innovative healthcare delivery, meaning that we must keep abreast of changes informed by current research, taking on board change for the better for our neonates and families within an evidence-based approach.

Finally, a consistent message that has been threaded throughout the book is the need to observe and check local practices. This book provides *general* principles taken from recent literature and/or national guidance, where applicable. However, we must always consider these general principles within the context of our own unit policies and the specifics of practice that have been agreed locally.

Knowledge to support safe and effective clinical practice is essential. This book aims to support knowledge for practice and serve as a bedside companion. The author welcomes any feedback and comments to guide future editions and to ensure the book content is tailored to the needs of it's audience.

Julia Petty
j.petty@herts.ac.uk

Acknowledgements

The author would like to thank the staff of the neonatal unit at the Royal London NHS Trust, Barts Health for their continuing support during her years there as link lecturer. The feedback and clinical knowledge gained from them has undoubtedly informed many of the key components of the book content.

Index

Printed by Printforce, the Netherlands